# Slow Cooker Dog Food Cookbook

*Elevate Your Dog's Health with Vet-Approved, Homemade Recipes Packed with Nutritious Ingredients Your Best Friend Will Love | Includes Tips for Busy Dog Owners*

Gisélle Rayne

© Copyright 2024 by GISÉLLE RAYNE- All rights reserved.

This document provides exact and reliable information regarding the topic and issues covered. The publication is sold with the idea that the publisher is not required to render accounting, officially permitted or otherwise qualified services. If advice is necessary, legal, or professional, a practiced individual in the profession should be ordered.

From a Declaration of Principles which was accepted and approved equally by a Committee of the American Bar Association and a Committee of Publishers and Associations.

In no way is it legal to reproduce, duplicate, or transmit any part of this document in either electronic means or printed format. Recording of this publication is prohibited, and any storage of this document is not allowed unless with written permission from the publisher. All rights reserved.

The information provided herein is stated to be truthful and consistent, in that any liability, in terms of inattention or otherwise, by any usage or abuse of any policies, processes, or Instructions contained within is the solitary and utter responsibility of the recipient reader. Under no circumstances will any legal responsibility or blame be held against the publisher for any reparation, damages, or monetary loss due to the information herein, either directly or indirectly.

Respective authors own all copyrights not held by the publisher.

The information herein is solely offered for informational purposes and is universal. The presentation of the information is without a contract or any guaranteed assurance.

The trademarks that are used are without any consent, and the publication of the trademark is without permission or backing by the trademark owner. All trademarks and brands within this book are for clarifying purposes only and are owned by the owners themselves, not affiliated with this document.

*In memory of my sweet and beloved Chlòe.*

# TABLE OF CONTENT

**INTRODUCTION** ........................................................................................................................ 5
   1. Introduction to Slow Cooking .......................................................................................... 5
   1.1 Differences Between Kibble and Homemade Meals ..................................................... 5
**CHAPTER 1: HEALTH BENEFITS** ............................................................................................ 6
   1.1 General Well-Being ....................................................................................................... 6
   1.1.1 Disease Prevention ................................................................................................... 6
   1.1.2 Importance of Hydration ........................................................................................... 7
**CHAPTER 2: ADVANTAGES OF SLOW COOKING** .................................................................. 9
   2.1 Preservation of Nutrients .............................................................................................. 9
   2.1.1 Comparison of Different Techniques ....................................................................... 9
   2.1.2 Improvement of Digestibility ................................................................................... 10
   2.2 Palatability .................................................................................................................. 10
**CHAPTER 3: ESSENTIAL INGREDIENTS FOR YOUR DOG'S HEALTH** ............................... 11
   3.1 List of Key Ingredients and Their Benefits ................................................................. 11
   3.2 List of Prohibited Ingredients and Why ...................................................................... 12
   3.3 Vegetables and Grains ............................................................................................... 13
   3.4 Fruits, Supplements, and Oils .................................................................................... 13
**CHAPTER 4: STORAGE AND SERVING TIPS** ........................................................................ 14
   4.1 Proper Storage Techniques ........................................................................................ 14
   4.2 Convenient Portioning ................................................................................................ 15
   4.3 Serving Tips ................................................................................................................ 16
   4.4 Food Safety Considerations ....................................................................................... 16
**CHAPTER 5: CURRENT TRENDS IN CANINE NUTRITION (2024)** ....................................... 17
   5.1 Innovations ................................................................................................................. 17
   5.1.1 Recent Studies ....................................................................................................... 17
   5.2 Eco-Sustainable Ingredients ...................................................................................... 17
   5.3 Diet Personalization ................................................................................................... 17
   5.4 Technology and Nutrition ........................................................................................... 17
**CHAPTER 6: SLOW COOKER RECIPES FOR DOGS** ............................................................ 18
**CHICKEN RECIPES** ................................................................................................................. 18
**TURKEY RECIPES** .................................................................................................................. 25
**BEEF RECIPES** ....................................................................................................................... 32
**LAMB RECIPES** ...................................................................................................................... 39
**PORK RECIPES** ...................................................................................................................... 46
**EGG RECIPES** ........................................................................................................................ 53
**LIVER RECIPES** ...................................................................................................................... 60
**HEART RECIPES** .................................................................................................................... 67
**SALMON RECIPES** ................................................................................................................. 74
**CODE RECIPES** ...................................................................................................................... 81
**TUNA RECIPES** ....................................................................................................................... 88
**SARDINE RECIPES** ................................................................................................................. 95
**TROUT RECIPES** .................................................................................................................. 102
**BONUS** .................................................................................................................................. 109
**COOKING MEASUREMENT TABLE** .................................................................................... 110
**CONCLUSIONS** ..................................................................................................................... 111

# Introduction

## 1. Introduction to Slow Cooking

Slow cooking is a technique that uses low temperatures and extended cooking times to prepare meals. Initially popular in human cuisine, this method is gaining traction in dog food preparation due to its numerous benefits. One of the primary advantages of slow cooking is its ability to preserve essential nutrients in food. This is particularly important for ensuring a balanced and nutrient-rich diet for dogs. Additionally, slow cooking enhances the digestibility of food, making nutrient absorption easier and reducing the risk of digestive issues. Slow cooking also allows for the preparation of fresh and customized meals using natural, high-quality ingredients. This helps to avoid preservatives and additives commonly found in commercial dog foods. Finally, slow-cooked foods develop richer and more intense flavors, making meals more appealing even to the pickiest dogs.

In summary, slow cooking offers an excellent way to prepare healthy and tasty meals for dogs, significantly contributing to their overall well-being and long-term health.

## 1.1 Differences Between Kibble and Homemade Meals

Commercial kibble is a common choice for dog feeding due to its convenience and balanced formulation. However, it can contain low-quality ingredients, artificial preservatives, and meat by-products. The high-temperature production process can degrade some nutrients, and some dogs may develop allergies to common kibble ingredients.

On the other hand, homemade meals offer complete control over the ingredients used, allowing for the selection of fresh, high-quality components. This customization can meet the specific needs of the dog, considering factors such as age, breed, and health conditions. The freshness of the ingredients also enhances the palatability of meals, making them more appetizing. Preparing meals at home requires time and a good understanding of the dog's nutritional needs, but with proper planning and consultation, it is possible to ensure a complete and balanced diet.

Overall, homemade meals offer superior nutrition and customization that kibble often cannot match, making them an excellent choice for owners who want the best for their dogs.

# Chapter 1: Health Benefits

## 1.1 General Well-Being

The benefits of a balanced, high-quality diet for dogs are numerous and impact various aspects of their health and well-being. Adopting a diet based on homemade meals prepared using the slow cooking technique can significantly improve your dog's life, ensuring optimal nutrition and helping to prevent many common diseases.
**Coat and Skin** A healthy and balanced diet is immediately reflected in the dog's coat and skin. The fresh and natural ingredients used in homemade meals, such as fish rich in omega-3 fatty acids, lean meat, and vitamin-rich vegetables, provide the essential nutrients necessary to keep the coat shiny and the skin healthy. Omega-3 fatty acids, in particular, have anti-inflammatory properties that help reduce skin irritations and improve overall skin health. The use of natural oils like coconut oil and fish oil can further contribute to improving coat quality and preventing common skin issues such as dryness, itching, and dermatitis.**Energy**
Homemade meals prepared using slow cooking offer a stable and long-lasting energy supply, thanks to the combination of high-quality proteins, complex carbohydrates, and healthy fats. Lean proteins, such as those from chicken and turkey, are essential for maintaining muscle mass and providing long-term energy. Complex carbohydrates from ingredients like brown rice and sweet potatoes release energy slowly, avoiding blood sugar spikes and keeping the dog active and alert throughout the day. Additionally, healthy fats present in ingredients like avocado (in moderate amounts and without the seed) and nuts (without xylitol) are essential for energy production and cellular health.
Disease Prevention
A balanced and nutrient-rich diet is one of the fundamental pillars for disease prevention. Homemade meals allow for the inclusion of specific ingredients that can help prevent common conditions in dogs, such as obesity, diabetes, heart disease, and joint diseases. For example, the inclusion of natural antioxidants from fresh fruits and vegetables helps combat free radicals and reduce the risk of developing tumors. Fiber-rich foods, such as pumpkin and carrots, improve digestion and contribute to intestinal health, preventing issues like constipation and gastrointestinal infections. Moreover, a diet free from artificial additives and preservatives reduces the risk of allergic reactions and food intolerances, ensuring a strong and responsive immune system.

### 1.1.1 Disease Prevention

Disease prevention in dogs is essential for ensuring a long and healthy life. A proper diet, combined with regular veterinary care and an active lifestyle, can significantly reduce the risk of many common conditions. Adopting a diet based on homemade meals prepared using the slow cooking technique can positively impact your dog's health in various ways.
**Immune System and Inflammation** A nutrient-rich diet is crucial for supporting the dog's immune system. Ingredients such as fatty fish, rich in omega-3 fatty acids, and leafy green vegetables, rich in antioxidants, help reduce inflammation and improve immune response. A strong immune system is the first line of defense against infections and chronic diseases, helping to keep the dog healthy and active.
**Cardiovascular Health** Heart health is another aspect that can greatly benefit from a well-balanced diet. Ingredients like salmon, nuts, and fish oil, which are rich in omega-3 fatty acids, help maintain cholesterol levels and improve blood circulation. The inclusion of natural antioxidants, such as those found in berries, helps prevent the oxidation of LDL cholesterol, thereby reducing the risk of heart disease.

### Joint Health

Ingredients rich in anti-inflammatory nutrients, such as turmeric and ginger, can help keep your dog's joints healthy and flexible. These ingredients can be easily incorporated into homemade meals, offering an added benefit compared to commercial diets. Slow cooking also allows for the extraction and preservation of vital nutrients from foods, such as collagen from bones, which is essential for joint health.

## Diabetes Prevention

A balanced diet with controlled amounts of complex carbohydrates and lean proteins can help prevent diabetes in dogs. Low-glycemic foods, such as sweet potatoes and brown rice, release glucose slowly into the bloodstream, avoiding spikes in blood sugar and helping to maintain stable blood sugar levels. This is particularly important for dogs predisposed to diabetes or those showing signs of insulin resistance.

## Cancer Prevention

Antioxidants found in fresh fruits and vegetables, such as blueberries and carrots, help combat free radicals that can cause cellular damage and lead to cancer development. Slow cooking preserves these essential nutrients, providing a diet rich in anti-cancer compounds that can help prevent tumor growth.
Investing time and resources in preparing healthy and balanced meals is an act of love that your dog will appreciate, reciprocating with a longer, healthier, and happier life.

## 1.1.2 Importance of Hydration

Hydration is essential for a dog's health and the proper functioning of all bodily systems. Water makes up about 60-70% of a dog's body weight and performs vital functions such as regulating body temperature, transporting nutrients, and eliminating toxins.
**Body Temperature Regulation** Dogs dissipate heat primarily through panting and sweating from their paws. Water is fundamental in this process, helping to keep body temperature within safe limits. During periods of intense heat or after physical activity, proper hydration is crucial to prevent heat stroke, a dangerous condition that can have severe consequences.
**Nutrient Transport** Water facilitates the transport of nutrients within the body. Nutrients absorbed from the intestines are dissolved in water and transported through the blood to all cells. This process is essential for maintaining optimal cellular functions and ensuring that every part of the body receives the necessary nutrients to function properly.
**Elimination of Toxins** Adequate hydration is crucial for the proper functioning of the kidneys, which are responsible for filtering the blood and eliminating toxins through urine. Without a sufficient amount of water, the kidneys cannot function properly, increasing the risk of toxin buildup in the body, which can lead to long-term health issues.

## Lubrication of Joints and Tissues

Water is an essential component of synovial fluid, which lubricates the joints, allowing for smooth movements and reducing friction. This is particularly important for older dogs or those with joint issues, such as arthritis. Additionally, water helps keep body tissues hydrated, including those in the eyes, mouth, and nose.

## How to Keep Your Dog Hydrated

Ensuring your dog stays hydrated requires attention and awareness. It's important to always provide access to fresh, clean water, changing it regularly. During hot months or after physical exercise, make sure your dog drinks regularly to replace lost fluids. Incorporating water-rich foods into their diet, such as fresh fruits and vegetables, can help increase their water intake.

## Signs of Dehydration and How to Prevent It

Recognizing the signs of dehydration is crucial for timely intervention. Common symptoms include dry and sticky gums, sunken eyes, lethargy, and loss of skin elasticity. To check for hydration, you can perform the skin pinch test: gently lift the skin on the dog's back; if it doesn't immediately return to place, the dog might be dehydrated. Ensuring constant access to fresh water, especially in hot conditions or during intense activity, is the best way to prevent dehydration.

Monitoring your dog's hydration is an essential act of care that can significantly impact their health and well-being.

# Chapter 2: Advantages of Slow Cooking

## 2.1 Preservation of Nutrients

Slow cooking is a technique that preserves the vital nutrients in food, essential for a healthy and balanced diet for dogs. By using moderate temperatures and extended cooking times, this technique minimizes the loss of vitamins, minerals, and other nutritional components.
**Vitamins and Minerals** Slow cooking helps maintain the vitamins and minerals crucial for a dog's health. Moderate temperatures prevent thermal degradation, preserving nutrients like vitamin C and B-complex vitamins.
**Digestive Enzymes** Digestive enzymes, necessary for the breakdown and absorption of nutrients, are better preserved due to the low temperatures of slow cooking, facilitating efficient digestion.
**Antioxidants** Antioxidants, which protect cells from damage caused by free radicals, are better preserved with slow cooking. This helps prevent chronic diseases and supports the immune system.
**Essential Amino Acids** Slow cooking preserves the integrity of essential amino acids, fundamental for building and maintaining body tissues, ensuring high-quality proteins for muscle growth and tissue repair.
Essential Fatty Acids
Essential fatty acids, such as omega-3 and omega-6, are protected from thermal degradation, maintaining a high content of beneficial fats for the health of the dog's skin and coat.
Dietary Fiber
Fiber, essential for digestive health, is better preserved with slow cooking, promoting good intestinal motility and preventing constipation.

## 2.1.1 Comparison of Different Techniques

When it comes to preparing meals for dogs, it is essential to understand the differences between various cooking techniques. Slow cooking stands out for its unique ability to preserve nutrients and improve food quality compared to other traditional cooking methods.
**High-Temperature Cooking** High-temperature cooking methods, such as frying, grilling, and boiling, are quick but often aggressive. These techniques can cause significant nutrient loss, particularly water-soluble vitamins like vitamin C and B vitamins. Additionally, high temperatures can denature proteins and reduce the bioavailability of some essential minerals. Frying, in particular, can introduce harmful trans fats, further compromising the nutritional quality of the meal.
**Steaming** Steaming is a gentler technique compared to high-temperature cooking. It allows for better nutrient preservation since boiling water does not directly contact the food. However, steaming can still result in the loss of some heat-sensitive vitamins, although to a lesser extent than boiling.
**Baking** Baking is a versatile technique that can be used at various temperatures. When performed at moderate temperatures, it can preserve nutrients better than high-temperature cooking. However, as with other methods, prolonged heat exposure can still degrade vitamins and minerals.

### Slow Cooking

Slow cooking, unlike the techniques mentioned above, uses low temperatures over extended periods. This approach allows for the best preservation of essential nutrients, such as water-soluble vitamins, amino acids, and essential fatty acids. Slow cooking maintains the structure of the food, improving digestibility and nutrient bioavailability. Additionally, the low temperature minimizes the formation of harmful compounds, such as acrylamides, which can form during high-temperature cooking.

The comparison of these techniques clearly demonstrates that slow cooking is the optimal choice for preparing highly nutritious meals for dogs, ensuring maximum preservation of essential nutrients and minimizing nutrient degradation.

## 2.1.2 Improvement of Digestibility

The digestibility of food is crucial in a dog's diet as it directly impacts the absorption of essential nutrients. Slow cooking significantly improves digestibility compared to other cooking techniques due to its ability to gradually break down proteins, making them more easily digestible. Proteins, essential for building and repairing tissues, are gently denatured, facilitating the action of digestive enzymes and improving the assimilation of essential amino acids.

Additionally, slow cooking better preserves the dietary fiber found in vegetables and grains, which is fundamental for digestive health, regulating intestinal transit, and maintaining a healthy gut flora. This cooking method also allows for a better breakdown of complex carbohydrates, increasing glucose availability and providing a steady and easily assimilable energy supply, keeping blood sugar levels stable.

Slow cooking reduces antinutrients present in some foods, improving the bioavailability of essential minerals such as iron and calcium. Moreover, it better preserves digestive enzymes, making nutrient assimilation more efficient for the dog. Finally, slow cooking softens muscle fibers and connective tissue in protein foods, making chewing and digestion easier, particularly beneficial for elderly dogs or those with dental issues.

## 2.2 Palatability

Ensuring that dogs enjoy their meals is essential for their well-being. The slow cooking technique, with its gentle approach, enhances the natural flavors of the ingredients without relying on artificial flavors or additives. By using low temperatures and prolonged cooking times, it promotes the development of rich and complex flavor profiles.

By cooking gradually, the ingredients retain their natural juices. This method prevents excessive drying of the food, ensuring a succulent and pleasant texture to chew. Animal proteins become more tender and flavorful, while vegetables and grains reveal all their aromatic notes, making the meal more delicious and stimulating the dog's appetite.

Combining different ingredients during cooking allows for the creation of harmonious and balanced dishes, with aromas that blend slowly to create irresistible flavors. This not only makes meals more appealing but also helps mask any supplements or medications added to the dog's diet, ensuring they are consumed without difficulty.

Additionally, this method maintains a soft and uniform texture of the food, facilitating chewing and digestion, particularly useful for elderly dogs or those with dental issues. It ensures that every bite is easily chewable, improving the overall dining experience for the dog.

# Chapter 3: Essential Ingredients for Your Dog's Health

## 3.1 List of Key Ingredients and Their Benefits

### Proteins

Proteins are a fundamental component of a dog's diet, essential for growth, tissue repair, and muscle mass maintenance. Proteins provide amino acids, the building blocks of cells, necessary for numerous biological functions, including the synthesis of enzymes, hormones, and antibodies. A diet rich in high-quality proteins supports a strong immune system, promotes a shiny coat and healthy skin, and contributes to the dog's overall vitality. Protein sources can include meat, fish, eggs, and organs, each offering a unique profile of essential amino acids and nutrients.

### Meat

| Food | Nutrients | Benefits |
|---|---|---|
| Chicken | Lean proteins, essential amino acids, B vitamins, phosphorus, selenium | Muscle growth, tissue repair |
| Turkey | Lean proteins, B6 and B12 vitamins, niacin, zinc | Digestion, immune system support |
| Beef | Proteins, iron, zinc, B12 vitamin | Red blood cell formation, general health |
| Lamb | Proteins, healthy fats | Beneficial for dogs with food sensitivities |
| Pork | Proteins, B1, B3, B6, B12 vitamins, iron, zinc | General health, immune function |
| Eggs | Proteins, vitamins, minerals | Coat and skin health |
| Liver | Vitamin A, iron, B vitamins | Blood health, immune function |
| Heart | Taurine, proteins | Cardiac health, muscle function |

### Fish

| Food | Nutrients | Benefits |
|---|---|---|
| Salmon | Omega-3 fatty acids, proteins | Skin and coat health, reduction of inflammation, improved cognitive function |
| Cod | Lean proteins, low fat content, vitamins, minerals | General health, low calorie content |
| Tuna | Proteins, omega-3 fatty acids | Cardiovascular health |
| Sardines | Calcium, vitamin D, omega-3 fatty acids | Bone and joint health |
| Trout | Proteins, essential fatty acids | Healthy skin, shiny coat |

## 3.2 List of Prohibited Ingredients and Why

### Meat

| Food | Dangerous Nutrients or Components | Reason |
|---|---|---|
| Raw pork | Potential presence of parasites | Risk of infection from trichinosis and other parasites |
| Cooked bones | Fragility | Can splinter and cause internal injuries |
| Liver* | High vitamin A content | Can cause vitamin A toxicity if consumed in excess |
| Bacon | High fat and salt content | Can cause pancreatitis and gastrointestinal issues |

**Note on liver:** Liver is a nutrient-rich food but must be given in moderation. High vitamin A content can cause toxicity if consumed in excess.

### Fish

| Food | Dangerous Nutrients or Components | Reason |
|---|---|---|
| Raw fish | Potential presence of thiaminase | Thiaminase destroys vitamin B1, causing deficiencies |
| Fish with bones | Bones | Can cause choking or internal injuries |
| Canned tuna | High mercury content | Risk of mercury toxicity |
| Pufferfish | Tetrodotoxin | Extremely toxic and potentially lethal |

### Other Dangerous Ingredients

| Food | Dangerous Nutrients or Components | Reason |
|---|---|---|
| Onions and garlic | Thiosulfate | Can cause hemolytic anemia in dogs |
| Chocolate | Theobromine | Highly toxic, can cause poisoning |
| Grapes and raisins | Unidentified components | Can cause acute renal failure |
| Avocado | Persin | Toxic for dogs, can cause gastrointestinal issues |
| Macadamia nuts | Unidentified toxic components | Can cause weakness, depression, and vomiting |
| Artificial sweeteners | Xylitol | Can cause hypoglycemia and liver failure |
| Alcohol | Ethanol | Can cause poisoning with severe symptoms |
| Coffee and tea | Caffeine | Can cause hyperactivity, tremors, and poisoning |
| Coconut | High potassium content | Can cause heart rhythm abnormalities |
| Yeast dough | Fermentation and gas production | Can cause bloating and gastric torsion |
| Nuts | High fat content | Can cause pancreatitis and digestive disorders |

## 3.3 Vegetables and Grains

Vegetables and grains are essential components of a balanced diet for dogs, providing a wide range of nutrients necessary for their overall well-being. Incorporating a variety of these foods into your dog's diet can improve digestion, provide sustainable energy, and support immune and cardiovascular health.

Vegetables offer a natural source of vitamins, minerals, and fiber, crucial for maintaining digestive health and preventing long-term health issues. For example, carrots and sweet potatoes are excellent sources of beta-carotene and vitamin A, essential for eye and skin health. Broccoli and spinach, rich in antioxidants, vitamins, and minerals, boost the immune system and support bone health.

Grains such as brown rice and oats provide complex carbohydrates that help maintain stable energy levels in dogs. These foods are also rich in fiber, supporting digestion and helping to maintain a healthy body weight. Quinoa and millet, in addition to being easily digestible, offer additional proteins and essential minerals like magnesium and iron, vital for muscle and nerve function.

### Vegetable Table

| Food | Nutrients | Benefits |
| --- | --- | --- |
| Carrots | Beta-carotene, vitamin A, fiber | Eye health, immune system support |
| Spinach | Vitamins A, C, K, iron, antioxidants | General health, immune support |
| Pumpkin | Fiber, vitamin A, potassium | Digestive health, regulation of bowel movements |
| Broccoli | Vitamins C, K, fiber, potassium | Immune support, bone health |
| Sweet Potatoes | Vitamin A, fiber, potassium | Digestive support, skin health |
| Zucchini | Vitamin C, manganese, fiber | Digestive support, general health |
| Cucumbers | Vitamin K, antioxidants | Hydration, low calorie |
| Green Beans | Vitamins A, C, K, fiber, iron | Digestive support, low calorie |
| Bell Peppers | Vitamins A, C | Immune support, skin health |
| Cauliflower | Vitamin C, fiber, antioxidants | Digestive support, immune support |
| Kale | Vitamins A, C, K, calcium, iron | Bone health, immune support |
| Peas | Protein, fiber, vitamins A, B, C, K | Energy, digestive support |
| Lettuce | Water, fiber, vitamins A, C | Hydration, digestive support |
| Beets | Fiber, vitamin C, potassium | Skin and coat health, digestive support |

### Grains Table

| Food | Nutrients | Benefits |
| --- | --- | --- |
| Brown Rice | Easily digestible carbohydrates, fiber | Energy, digestive support |
| Oats | Soluble fiber, protein, iron | Blood sugar level maintenance, digestive support |
| Quinoa | Protein, fiber, iron, magnesium | Energy, muscular and nervous system support |
| Barley | Fiber, B vitamins, selenium | Digestive support, heart health |
| Millet | Carbohydrates, magnesium, phosphorus | Energy, bone support |

## 3.4 Fruits, Supplements, and Oils

Fruits, supplements, and oils are essential components of a balanced diet for dogs. These ingredients provide vitamins, minerals, and essential fatty acids that support the overall health of your dog, helping to improve the immune system, skin and coat health, and heart function. It is important to carefully choose these foods to ensure your dog receives all necessary nutrients without risk of overdose or deficiencies.

## Fruits Table

| Food | Nutrients | Benefits |
|---|---|---|
| Apples | Vitamin C, fiber, antioxidants | Digestive health, immune support |
| Blueberries | Antioxidants, fiber, vitamins C and K | Brain health, immune support |
| Bananas | Vitamin B6, vitamin C, potassium | Energy, muscle support |
| Strawberries | Vitamin C, fiber, antioxidants | Heart health, immune support |
| Watermelon | Vitamin A, vitamin C, antioxidants | Hydration, low calorie |
| Oranges | Vitamin C, fiber | Immune support, digestive health |
| Pears | Fiber, vitamin C, vitamin K | Digestive support, bone health |

## Supplements Table

| Supplement | Nutrients | Benefits |
|---|---|---|
| Omega-3 | Essential fatty acids | Skin and coat health, heart function |
| Glucosamine | Amino sugar | Joint support, arthritis prevention |
| Probiotics | Beneficial bacteria | Digestive health, immune support |
| Multivitamins | Various vitamins and minerals | General health support, prevention of deficiencies |
| Chondroitin | Polysaccharide complex | Joint support, arthritis prevention |

## Oils Table

| Oil | Nutrients | Benefits |
|---|---|---|
| Fish oil | Omega-3, DHA, EPA | Skin and coat health, heart function |
| Coconut oil | Medium-chain fatty acids | Digestive health, skin and coat support |
| Olive oil | Vitamin E, antioxidants | Cardiovascular support, skin health |
| Flaxseed oil | Omega-3, alpha-linolenic acid | Skin health, immune support |

# Chapter 4: Storage and Serving Tips

## 4.1 Proper Storage Techniques

To ensure that homemade dog food remains safe and nutritious, it is essential to follow proper storage techniques. Correct storage not only preserves essential nutrients but also prevents the growth of harmful bacteria and mold that could jeopardize your dog's health. Here are some fundamental guidelines for storing homemade dog food.
**Storage in Airtight Containers** Using airtight containers is crucial to prevent exposure to air, which can accelerate food spoilage. Glass or BPA-free plastic containers are ideal for keeping food fresh. These containers help preserve food quality and prevent external contamination.
**Refrigeration** Homemade dog food, intended for consumption within a few days, should be stored in the refrigerator. The refrigerator temperature should consistently be kept below 4°C (40°F). It is advisable to label each container with the preparation date to monitor food freshness. Refrigerated food should be consumed within 3-5 days to ensure maximum safety and quality.

## Freezing

For long-term storage, freezing is the best option. Use sturdy freezer bags or freezer-safe containers. It is important to label each container with the preparation date and type of food. Frozen food should be consumed within 3-6 months to ensure maximum freshness and quality.

## Thawing and Heating Instructions

Thawing frozen food should be done in the refrigerator, not at room temperature, to prevent bacterial growth. Alternatively, a microwave can be used for quick thawing, but make sure the food does not become too hot before serving it to the dog. Warming the food to room temperature or slightly warm is ideal to avoid burns and ensure the dog can consume it comfortably.
By following these storage techniques, you can ensure that homemade dog food remains safe, nutritious, and tasty for a longer period, contributing to the overall well-being of your four-legged friend.

## 4.2 Convenient Portioning

Proper portioning of homemade dog food is essential to ensure that your furry friend receives the right amount of nutrients without any waste. Here are some tips to make portioning simple and convenient.

## Measuring Portions

To determine the appropriate amount of food for your dog, consider their size, age, activity level, and health condition. Using a kitchen scale to measure portions accurately is recommended. Alternatively, you can use specific measuring cups and spoons for food.

## Pre-Portioning

Pre-portioning food into individual servings helps maintain freshness and simplifies daily meals. You can use freezer bags or airtight containers to divide food into daily or weekly portions. Label each portion with the preparation date and type of food for optimal management.

## Labeling

Label each container or bag with details such as the preparation date, quantity, and type of food. This helps track inventory and ensures that older food is used first. This labeling system is crucial to avoid waste and ensure the food remains safe and nutritious.

## Using Suitable Containers

Choose high-quality airtight containers to store pre-portioned food. Glass or BPA-free plastic containers are ideal for keeping food fresh and preventing contamination. Ensure the containers are suitable for both refrigeration and freezing.

## FIFO System

Implementing the "First In, First Out" (FIFO) system is an effective practice for managing food supplies. This system ensures that the food prepared first is consumed first, reducing the risk of spoilage and waste.

## 4.3 Serving Tips

Serving homemade dog food properly is essential to ensure your furry friend gets the maximum nutritional benefit from each meal. Here are some practical tips to ensure the food is served safely and effectively.
**Food Temperature** Before serving the food to your dog, make sure it is at room temperature or slightly warm. Food that is too hot can cause burns, while food that is too cold might be less appealing to the dog. Warming the food in the microwave for a few seconds or letting it sit at room temperature for a while can help achieve the ideal temperature.
**Clean Bowls** Always keep your dog's food and water bowls clean. Wash the bowls with hot, soapy water after each meal to prevent the buildup of bacteria and food residues. Using stainless steel or ceramic bowls, which are easier to clean and less likely to harbor bacteria than plastic ones, is recommended.
**Proper Portions** Ensure you serve adequate portions based on your dog's size, age, activity level, and health conditions. Using precise measuring tools like measuring cups or kitchen scales can help ensure your dog receives the correct amount of food.
**Meal Routine** Establish a regular meal routine for your dog by serving meals at the same time each day. This helps maintain your dog's metabolism in balance and can improve digestion. Additionally, a regular routine can help prevent behavioral issues related to feeding.
**Adding Supplements** If your dog needs dietary supplements, make sure to mix them thoroughly into the food to ensure even intake. Consult with your veterinarian to determine which supplements are necessary and the appropriate amount to give.
**Monitoring Consumption** Observe your dog's behavior during meals. If you notice your dog eating too quickly, consider using a slow-feeder bowl to slow down the eating pace. This can help prevent digestive issues like bloating and improve digestion.

## 4.4 Food Safety Considerations

Food safety is a crucial aspect of preparing homemade dog food. To ensure the health of your furry friend, it is essential to follow strict hygienic practices. Here are some essential guidelines based on official and reliable sources.
**Safe Handling of Ingredients** Wash your hands thoroughly with soap and water before and after handling your dog's food, especially if handling raw meat. Utensils and surfaces used for preparing the food should be washed and disinfected thoroughly after each use. Use separate cutting boards for meat and other ingredients to avoid cross-contamination.
**Proper Cooking** Meat and fish should be cooked to safe temperatures to kill any harmful bacteria. Meat should reach an internal temperature of at least 165°F (74°C) to ensure it is safe to consume. Avoid serving raw or undercooked meat, as it may contain pathogens that could cause foodborne illnesses in dogs.

# Chapter 5: Current Trends in Canine Nutrition (2024)

## 5.1 Innovations

Innovations in canine nutrition are emerging as a response to the growing health and wellness needs of pets. Key trends include:
- **Functional Foods:** The inclusion of functional ingredients such as prebiotics and probiotics to improve gut health, and natural ingredients like mushrooms, turmeric, and ginger to support the immune system and reduce inflammation.
- **High-Quality Protein Integration:** High-protein diets are gaining popularity for their ability to maintain muscle mass and promote healthy weight loss.

### 5.1.1 Recent Studies
Scientific research continues to explore new frontiers in pet nutrition:
- **Gut-Brain Axis Study:** The connection between gut health and mental well-being in dogs is being extensively studied. Foods rich in prebiotic and probiotic fibers are essential for maintaining a healthy gut microbiome, which positively affects the dog's behavior and mood.
- **Omega-3 and Inflammation:** Recent studies have shown that omega-3 fatty acids, such as EPA and DHA, can reduce inflammatory markers in dogs, improving joint health and reducing symptoms of osteoarthritis.

## 5.2 Eco-Sustainable Ingredients
The focus on environmental sustainability has led to an increased use of eco-sustainable ingredients in dog nutrition:
- **Plant-Based Ingredients:** Adopting diets more oriented towards plant-based ingredients not only offers nutritional benefits but also reduces environmental impact. For example, the use of plant proteins such as lentils, peas, and quinoa is becoming more common.
- **Sustainable Packaging:** Many companies are transitioning to recyclable and compostable packaging to reduce waste and promote responsible consumption practices.

## 5.3 Diet Personalization

- **Tailored Diets:** The rise in the use of personalized meal plans to meet the specific nutritional needs of each dog, considering factors such as age, breed, activity level, and health conditions.

## 5.4 Technology and Nutrition

- **Health Monitoring:** The use of technological devices to monitor the health and activity of dogs, helping owners optimize nutrition and exercise.
- **Nutrition Apps:** The introduction of mobile applications that offer personalized diet advice and help plan meals.
SLOW COOKER COOKBOOK

# Chapter 6: Slow Cooker Recipes for Dogs

## Chicken Recipes

### Recipe 1: Chicken, Rice, and Veggies

**Ingredients (for 1 cup):**

- 1.6 oz boneless, skinless chicken breast, cubed
- 2 tbsp brown rice, rinsed
- 1/4 cup carrots, chopped
- 1/4 cup spinach, chopped
- 1/2 tsp flaxseed oil or fish oil (optional)
- 1 cup water
- A pinch of crushed eggshell (for calcium)

**Preparation Time:**

- **Prep Time**: 10 minutes
- **Cook Time**: 4 hours on low
- **Total Time**: 4 hours 10 minutes
- **Difficulty Level**: Easy

**Instructions:**

1. **Prepare the Ingredients**:
    - Cube the chicken breast.
    - Rinse the brown rice.
    - Chop the carrots and spinach.
2. **Combine in Slow Cooker**:
    - Place the chicken, brown rice, carrots, and spinach in the slow cooker.
    - Add 1 cup of water to ensure there is enough moisture.
    - Drizzle with flaxseed oil or fish oil (optional).
3. **Cook**:
    - Set the slow cooker to low and cook for 4 hours or until the chicken is fully cooked and the vegetables and rice are tender.
4. **Cool and Serve**:
    - Allow the mixture to cool to a safe temperature before serving.
    - Portion according to your dog's size and daily caloric needs.

## Nutritional Information (per serving):

| Nutrient | Quantity (per cup) | Daily Value (%) |
|---|---|---|
| Calories | 65 kcal | - |
| Protein | 1.2 oz (34.1 g) | 52.45% |
| Fat | 0.3 oz (8.9 g) | 13.71% |
| Carbohydrates | 0.6 oz (17.4 g) | 33.83% |
| Fiber | 0.02 oz (0.6 g) | 0.93% |

## Suggested Portions (Daily):

| Dog Size (lbs) | Low Activity | Moderate Activity | High Activity |
|---|---|---|---|
| 5 | 1/2 cup | 3/4 cup | 1 cup |
| 10 | 1 cup | 1 1/2 cups | 2 cups |
| 20 | 2 cups | 2 1/2 cups | 3 cups |
| 30 | 2 1/2 cups | 3 1/2 cups | 4 cups |
| 40 | 3 cups | 4 cups | 5 cups |
| 50 | 3 1/2 cups | 4 1/2 cups | 5 1/2 cups |
| 60 | 4 cups | 5 cups | 6 cups |
| 70 | 4 1/2 cups | 5 1/2 cups | 6 1/2 cups |
| 80 | 5 cups | 6 cups | 7 cups |
| 90 | 5 1/2 cups | 6 1/2 cups | 7 1/2 cups |
| 100 | 6 cups | 7 cups | 8 cups |

## Recipe 2: Chicken, Sweet Potatoes, and Green Beans

**Ingredients (for 1 cup):**

- 1.6 oz boneless, skinless chicken breast, cubed
- 2 tbsp quinoa, rinsed
- 1/4 cup sweet potatoes, diced
- 1/4 cup green beans, chopped
- 1/2 tsp olive oil or fish oil (optional)
- 1 cup water
- A pinch of crushed eggshell (for calcium)

**Preparation Time:**

- **Prep Time**: 10 minutes
- **Cook Time**: 4 hours on low
- **Total Time**: 4 hours 10 minutes
- **Difficulty Level**: Easy

**Instructions:**

1. **Prepare the Ingredients**:
    - Cube the chicken breast.
    - Rinse the quinoa.
    - Dice the sweet potatoes and chop the green beans.

2. **Combine in Slow Cooker**:
    - Place the chicken, quinoa, sweet potatoes, and green beans in the slow cooker.
    - Add 1 cup of water to ensure there is enough moisture.
    - Drizzle with olive oil or fish oil (optional).
3. **Cook**:
    - Set the slow cooker to low and cook for 4 hours or until the chicken is fully cooked and the vegetables and quinoa are tender.
4. **Cool and Serve**:
    - Allow the mixture to cool to a safe temperature before serving.
    - Portion according to your dog's size and daily caloric needs.

## Nutritional Information (per serving):

| Nutrient | Quantity (per cup) | Daily Value (%) |
|---|---|---|
| Calories | 143 kcal | - |
| Protein | 0.6 oz (17.5 g) | 50.92% |
| Fat | 0.07 oz (2.0 g) | 13.01% |
| Carbohydrates | 0.78 oz (22.4 g) | 36.07% |
| Fiber | 0.05 oz (1.3 g) | 1.33% |

## Suggested Portions (Daily):

| Dog Size (lbs) | Low Activity | Moderate Activity | High Activity |
|---|---|---|---|
| 5 | 1/2 cup | 3/4 cup | 1 cup |
| 10 | 1 cup | 1 1/2 cups | 2 cups |
| 20 | 2 cups | 2 1/2 cups | 3 cups |
| 30 | 2 1/2 cups | 3 1/2 cups | 4 cups |
| 40 | 3 cups | 4 cups | 5 cups |
| 50 | 3 1/2 cups | 4 1/2 cups | 5 1/2 cups |
| 60 | 4 cups | 5 cups | 6 cups |
| 70 | 4 1/2 cups | 5 1/2 cups | 6 1/2 cups |
| 80 | 5 cups | 6 cups | 7 cups |
| 90 | 5 1/2 cups | 6 1/2 cups | 7 1/2 cups |
| 100 | 6 cups | 7 cups | 8 cups |

## Recipe 3: Chicken, Rice, and Garden Veggies

**Ingredients (for 1 cup):**

- 1.6 oz boneless, skinless chicken breast, cubed
- 2 tbsp brown rice, rinsed
- 1/4 cup peas
- 1/4 cup broccoli, chopped
- 1/2 tsp flaxseed oil or fish oil (optional)
- 1 cup water
- A pinch of crushed eggshell (for calcium)

**Preparation Time:**

- **Prep Time**: 10 minutes
- **Cook Time**: 4 hours on low
- **Total Time**: 4 hours 10 minutes
- **Difficulty Level**: Easy

**Instructions:**

1. **Prepare the Ingredients**:
    - Cube the chicken breast.
    - Rinse the brown rice.
    - Chop the broccoli.
2. **Combine in Slow Cooker**:
    - Place the chicken, brown rice, peas, and broccoli in the slow cooker.
    - Add 1 cup of water to ensure there is enough moisture.
    - Drizzle with flaxseed oil or fish oil (optional).
3. **Cook**:
    - Set the slow cooker to low and cook for 4 hours or until the chicken is fully cooked and the vegetables and rice are tender.
4. **Cool and Serve**:
    - Allow the mixture to cool to a safe temperature before serving.
    - Portion according to your dog's size and daily caloric needs.

## Nutritional Information (per serving):

| Nutrient | Quantity (per cup) | Daily Value (%) |
|---|---|---|
| Calories | 179 kcal | - |
| Protein | 0.7 oz (21.1 g) | 46.11% |
| Fat | 0.04 oz (1.9 g) | 10.90% |
| Carbohydrates | 0.92 oz (26.4 g) | 42.99% |
| Fiber | 0.08 oz (2.2 g) | 2.16% |

## Suggested Portions (Daily):

| Dog Size (lbs) | Low Activity | Moderate Activity | High Activity |
|---|---|---|---|
| 5 | 1/2 cup | 3/4 cup | 1 cup |
| 10 | 1 cup | 1 1/2 cups | 2 cups |
| 20 | 2 cups | 2 1/2 cups | 3 cups |
| 30 | 2 1/2 cups | 3 1/2 cups | 4 cups |
| 40 | 3 cups | 4 cups | 5 cups |
| 50 | 3 1/2 cups | 4 1/2 cups | 5 1/2 cups |
| 60 | 4 cups | 5 cups | 6 cups |
| 70 | 4 1/2 cups | 5 1/2 cups | 6 1/2 cups |
| 80 | 5 cups | 6 cups | 7 cups |
| 90 | 5 1/2 cups | 6 1/2 cups | 7 1/2 cups |
| 100 | 6 cups | 7 cups | 8 cups |

## Recipe 4: Chicken, Rice, and Blueberry Delight

**Ingredients (for 1 cup):**

- 1.6 oz boneless, skinless chicken breast, cubed
- 2 tbsp brown rice, rinsed
- 1/4 cup peas
- 1/4 cup broccoli, chopped
- 1/4 cup blueberries
- 1/2 tsp flaxseed oil or fish oil (optional)
- 1 cup water
- A pinch of crushed eggshell (for calcium)

**Preparation Time:**

- **Prep Time**: 10 minutes
- **Cook Time**: 4 hours on low
- **Total Time**: 4 hours 10 minutes
- **Difficulty Level**: Easy

**Instructions:**

1. **Prepare the Ingredients**:
    - Cube the chicken breast.
    - Rinse the brown rice.
    - Chop the broccoli.
2. **Combine in Slow Cooker**:
    - Place the chicken, brown rice, peas, broccoli, and blueberries in the slow cooker.
    - Add 1 cup of water to ensure there is enough moisture.
    - Drizzle with flaxseed oil or fish oil (optional).
3. **Cook**:
    - Set the slow cooker to low and cook for 4 hours or until the chicken is fully cooked and the vegetables and rice are tender.
4. **Cool and Serve**:
    - Allow the mixture to cool to a safe temperature before serving.
    - Portion according to your dog's size and daily caloric needs.

## Nutritional Information (per serving):

| Nutrient | Quantity (per cup) | Daily Value (%) |
|---|---|---|
| Calories | 196 kcal | - |
| Protein | 0.64 oz (18.24 g) | 40.72% |
| Fat | 0.15 oz (4.35 g) | 9.72% |
| Carbohydrates | 0.75 oz (21.16 g) | 47.24% |
| Fiber | 0.08 oz (2.2 g) | 2.16% |

## Suggested Portions (Daily):

| Dog Size (lbs) | Low Activity | Moderate Activity | High Activity |
|---|---|---|---|
| 5 | 1/2 cup | 3/4 cup | 1 cup |
| 10 | 1 cup | 1 1/2 cups | 2 cups |
| 20 | 2 cups | 2 1/2 cups | 3 cups |
| 30 | 2 1/2 cups | 3 1/2 cups | 4 cups |
| 40 | 3 cups | 4 cups | 5 cups |
| 50 | 3 1/2 cups | 4 1/2 cups | 5 1/2 cups |
| 60 | 4 cups | 5 cups | 6 cups |
| 70 | 4 1/2 cups | 5 1/2 cups | 6 1/2 cups |
| 80 | 5 cups | 6 cups | 7 cups |
| 90 | 5 1/2 cups | 6 1/2 cups | 7 1/2 cups |
| 100 | 6 cups | 7 cups | 8 cups |

## Recipe 5: Chicken, Sweet Potato, and Apple Feast

**Ingredients (for 1 cup):**

- 1.6 oz boneless, skinless chicken breast, cubed
- 1/4 cup sweet potatoes, diced
- 1/4 cup green beans, chopped
- 1/4 cup apples, chopped
- 1/2 tsp olive oil or fish oil (optional)
- 1 cup water
- A pinch of crushed eggshell (for calcium)

**Preparation Time:**

- **Prep Time**: 10 minutes
- **Cook Time**: 4 hours on low
- **Total Time**: 4 hours 10 minutes
- **Difficulty Level**: Easy

**Instructions:**

1. **Prepare the Ingredients**:
   - Cube the chicken breast.
   - Dice the sweet potatoes.
   - Chop the green beans and apples.
2. **Combine in Slow Cooker**:
   - Place the chicken, sweet potatoes, green beans, and apples in the slow cooker.
   - Add 1 cup of water to ensure there is enough moisture.
   - Drizzle with olive oil or fish oil (optional).
3. **Cook**:
   - Set the slow cooker to low and cook for 4 hours or until the chicken is fully cooked and the vegetables are tender.

4. **Cool and Serve**:
    o Allow the mixture to cool to a safe temperature before serving.
    o Portion according to your dog's size and daily caloric needs.

## Nutritional Information (per serving):

| Nutrient | Quantity (per cup) | Daily Value (%) |
|---|---|---|
| Calories | 141 kcal | - |
| Protein | 0.64 oz (18.24 g) | 48.79% |
| Fat | 0.04 oz (1.72 g) | 12.17% |
| Carbohydrates | 0.55 oz (21.16 g) | 39.04% |
| Fiber | 0.06 oz (1.73 g) | 1.73% |

## Suggested Portions (Daily):

| Dog Size (lbs) | Low Activity | Moderate Activity | High Activity |
|---|---|---|---|
| 5 | 1/2 cup | 3/4 cup | 1 cup |
| 10 | 1 cup | 1 1/2 cups | 2 cups |
| 20 | 2 cups | 2 1/2 cups | 3 cups |
| 30 | 2 1/2 cups | 3 1/2 cups | 4 cups |
| 40 | 3 cups | 4 cups | 5 cups |
| 50 | 3 1/2 cups | 4 1/2 cups | 5 1/2 cups |
| 60 | 4 cups | 5 cups | 6 cups |
| 70 | 4 1/2 cups | 5 1/2 cups | 6 1/2 cups |
| 80 | 5 cups | 6 cups | 7 cups |
| 90 | 5 1/2 cups | 6 1/2 cups | 7 1/2 cups |
| 100 | 6 cups | 7 cups | 8 cups |

# Turkey Recipes

## Recipe 1: Turkey, Rice, and Veggie Medley

**Ingredients (for 1 cup):**

- 1.6 oz boneless, skinless turkey breast, cubed
- 2 tbsp brown rice, rinsed
- 1/4 cup carrots, chopped
- 1/4 cup spinach, chopped
- 1/2 tsp flaxseed oil or fish oil (optional)
- 1 cup water
- A pinch of crushed eggshell (for calcium)

**Preparation Time:**

- **Prep Time**: 10 minutes
- **Cook Time**: 4 hours on low
- **Total Time**: 4 hours 10 minutes
- **Difficulty Level**: Easy

**Instructions:**

1. **Prepare the Ingredients**:
   - Cube the turkey breast.
   - Rinse the brown rice.
   - Chop the carrots and spinach.
2. **Combine in Slow Cooker**:
   - Place the turkey, brown rice, carrots, and spinach in the slow cooker.
   - Add 1 cup of water to ensure there is enough moisture.
   - Drizzle with flaxseed oil or fish oil (optional).
3. **Cook**:
   - Set the slow cooker to low and cook for 4 hours or until the turkey is fully cooked and the vegetables and rice are tender.
4. **Cool and Serve**:
   - Allow the mixture to cool to a safe temperature before serving.
   - Portion according to your dog's size and daily caloric needs.

## Nutritional Information (per serving):

| Nutrient | Quantity (per cup) | Daily Value (%) |
|---|---|---|
| Calories | 133 kcal | - |
| Protein | 0.64 oz (18.22 g) | 52.04% |
| Fat | 0.03 oz (1.73 g) | 9.89% |
| Carbohydrates | 0.62 oz (17.98 g) | 38.07% |
| Fiber | 0.04 oz (1.09 g) | 1.09% |

## Suggested Portions (Daily):

| Dog Size (lbs) | Low Activity | Moderate Activity | High Activity |
|---|---|---|---|
| 5 | 1/2 cup | 3/4 cup | 1 cup |
| 10 | 1 cup | 1 1/2 cups | 2 cups |
| 20 | 2 cups | 2 1/2 cups | 3 cups |
| 30 | 2 1/2 cups | 3 1/2 cups | 4 cups |
| 40 | 3 cups | 4 cups | 5 cups |
| 50 | 3 1/2 cups | 4 1/2 cups | 5 1/2 cups |
| 60 | 4 cups | 5 cups | 6 cups |
| 70 | 4 1/2 cups | 5 1/2 cups | 6 1/2 cups |
| 80 | 5 cups | 6 cups | 7 cups |
| 90 | 5 1/2 cups | 6 1/2 cups | 7 1/2 cups |
| 100 | 6 cups | 7 cups | 8 cups |

## Recipe 2: Turkey, Quinoa, and Garden Greens Delight

**Ingredients (for 1 cup):**

- 1.6 oz boneless, skinless turkey breast, cubed
- 2 tbsp quinoa, rinsed
- 1/4 cup peas
- 1/4 cup broccoli, chopped
- 1/2 tsp flaxseed oil or fish oil (optional)
- 1 cup water
- A pinch of crushed eggshell (for calcium)

**Preparation Time:**

- **Prep Time**: 10 minutes
- **Cook Time**: 4 hours on low
- **Total Time**: 4 hours 10 minutes
- **Difficulty Level**: Easy

**Instructions:**

1. **Prepare the Ingredients**:
   - Cube the turkey breast.
   - Rinse the quinoa.
   - Chop the broccoli.
2. **Combine in Slow Cooker**:
   - Place the turkey, quinoa, peas, and broccoli in the slow cooker.
   - Add 1 cup of water to ensure there is enough moisture.
   - Drizzle with flaxseed oil or fish oil (optional).
3. **Cook**:
   - Set the slow cooker to low and cook for 4 hours or until the turkey is fully cooked and the vegetables and quinoa are tender.

4. **Cool and Serve**:
   o Allow the mixture to cool to a safe temperature before serving.
   o Portion according to your dog's size and daily caloric needs.

## Nutritional Information (per serving):

| Nutrient | Quantity (per cup) | Daily Value (%) |
|---|---|---|
| Calories | 147 kcal | - |
| Protein | 0.66 oz (19.09 g) | 53.03% |
| Fat | 0.03 oz (1.37 g) | 9.38% |
| Carbohydrates | 0.66 oz (20.47 g) | 37.59% |
| Fiber | 0.08 oz (2.40 g) | 2.40% |

## Suggested Portions (Daily):

| Dog Size (lbs) | Low Activity | Moderate Activity | High Activity |
|---|---|---|---|
| 5 | 1/2 cup | 3/4 cup | 1 cup |
| 10 | 1 cup | 1 1/2 cups | 2 cups |
| 20 | 2 cups | 2 1/2 cups | 3 cups |
| 30 | 2 1/2 cups | 3 1/2 cups | 4 cups |
| 40 | 3 cups | 4 cups | 5 cups |
| 50 | 3 1/2 cups | 4 1/2 cups | 5 1/2 cups |
| 60 | 4 cups | 5 cups | 6 cups |
| 70 | 4 1/2 cups | 5 1/2 cups | 6 1/2 cups |
| 80 | 5 cups | 6 cups | 7 cups |
| 90 | 5 1/2 cups | 6 1/2 cups | 7 1/2 cups |
| 100 | 6 cups | 7 cups | 8 cups |

## Recipe 3: Turkey, Sweet Potato, and Apple Medley

**Ingredients (for 1 cup):**

- 1.6 oz boneless, skinless turkey breast, cubed
- 1/4 cup sweet potatoes, diced
- 1/4 cup green beans, chopped
- 1/4 cup apples, chopped
- 1/2 tsp olive oil or fish oil (optional)
- 1 cup water
- A pinch of crushed eggshell (for calcium)

**Preparation Time:**

- **Prep Time**: 10 minutes
- **Cook Time**: 4 hours on low
- **Total Time**: 4 hours 10 minutes
- **Difficulty Level**: Easy

**Instructions:**

1. **Prepare the Ingredients:**
    - Cube the turkey breast.
    - Dice the sweet potatoes.
    - Chop the green beans and apples.
2. **Combine in Slow Cooker:**
    - Place the turkey, sweet potatoes, green beans, and apples in the slow cooker.
    - Add 1 cup of water to ensure there is enough moisture.
    - Drizzle with olive oil or fish oil (optional).
3. **Cook:**
    - Set the slow cooker to low and cook for 4 hours or until the turkey is fully cooked and the vegetables are tender.
4. **Cool and Serve:**
    - Allow the mixture to cool to a safe temperature before serving.
    - Portion according to your dog's size and daily caloric needs.

## Nutritional Information (per serving):

| Nutrient | Quantity (per cup) | Daily Value (%) |
| --- | --- | --- |
| Calories | 128 kcal | - |
| Protein | 0.63 oz (17.99 g) | 49.96% |
| Fat | 0.03 oz (1.12 g) | 8.83% |
| Carbohydrates | 0.75 oz (20.91 g) | 41.22% |
| Fiber | 0.06 oz (1.73 g) | 1.73% |

## Suggested Portions (Daily):

| Dog Size (lbs) | Low Activity | Moderate Activity | High Activity |
| --- | --- | --- | --- |
| 5 | 1/2 cup | 3/4 cup | 1 cup |
| 10 | 1 cup | 1 1/2 cups | 2 cups |
| 20 | 2 cups | 2 1/2 cups | 3 cups |
| 30 | 2 1/2 cups | 3 1/2 cups | 4 cups |
| 40 | 3 cups | 4 cups | 5 cups |
| 50 | 3 1/2 cups | 4 1/2 cups | 5 1/2 cups |
| 60 | 4 cups | 5 cups | 6 cups |
| 70 | 4 1/2 cups | 5 1/2 cups | 6 1/2 cups |
| 80 | 5 cups | 6 cups | 7 cups |
| 90 | 5 1/2 cups | 6 1/2 cups | 7 1/2 cups |
| 100 | 6 cups | 7 cups | 8 cups |

## Recipe 4: Turkey, Rice, and Blueberry Bliss (Revised)

**Ingredients (for 1 cup):**

- 1.6 oz boneless, skinless turkey breast, cubed
- 2 tbsp brown rice, rinsed
- 1/4 cup zucchini, chopped

- 1/4 cup blueberries
- 1/4 cup carrots, chopped
- 1/2 tsp olive oil or fish oil (optional)
- 1 cup water
- A pinch of crushed eggshell (for calcium)

**Preparation Time:**

- **Prep Time**: 10 minutes
- **Cook Time**: 4 hours on low
- **Total Time**: 4 hours 10 minutes
- **Difficulty Level**: Easy

**Instructions:**

1. **Prepare the Ingredients**:
    - Cube the turkey breast.
    - Rinse the brown rice.
    - Chop the zucchini and carrots.
    - Measure out the blueberries.
2. **Combine in Slow Cooker**:
    - Place the turkey, brown rice, zucchini, carrots, and blueberries in the slow cooker.
    - Add 1 cup of water to ensure there is enough moisture.
    - Drizzle with olive oil or fish oil (optional).
3. **Cook**:
    - Set the slow cooker to low and cook for 4 hours or until the turkey is fully cooked and the vegetables are tender.
4. **Cool and Serve**:
    - Allow the mixture to cool to a safe temperature before serving.
    - Portion according to your dog's size and daily caloric needs.

## Nutritional Information (per serving):

| Nutrient | Quantity (per cup) | Daily Value (%) |
| --- | --- | --- |
| Calories | 148 kcal | - |
| Protein | 0.63 oz (18.24 g) | 48.23% |
| Fat | 0.03 oz (1.31 g) | 8.68% |
| Carbohydrates | 0.80 oz (22.67 g) | 42.82% |
| Fiber | 0.05 oz (1.32 g) | 1.32% |

## Suggested Portions (Daily):

| Dog Size (lbs) | Low Activity | Moderate Activity | High Activity |
|---|---|---|---|
| 5 | 1/2 cup | 3/4 cup | 1 cup |
| 10 | 1 cup | 1 1/2 cups | 2 cups |
| 20 | 2 cups | 2 1/2 cups | 3 cups |
| 30 | 2 1/2 cups | 3 1/2 cups | 4 cups |
| 40 | 3 cups | 4 cups | 5 cups |
| 50 | 3 1/2 cups | 4 1/2 cups | 5 1/2 cups |
| 60 | 4 cups | 5 cups | 6 cups |
| 70 | 4 1/2 cups | 5 1/2 cups | 6 1/2 cups |
| 80 | 5 cups | 6 cups | 7 cups |
| 90 | 5 1/2 cups | 6 1/2 cups | 7 1/2 cups |
| 100 | 6 cups | 7 cups | 8 cups |

## Recipe 5: Turkey, Rice, and Pumpkin Feast

**Ingredients (for 1 cup):**

- 1.6 oz boneless, skinless turkey breast, cubed
- 2 tbsp brown rice, rinsed
- 1/4 cup pumpkin, cooked and mashed
- 1/4 cup peas
- 1/4 cup carrots, chopped
- 1/2 tsp olive oil or fish oil (optional)
- 1 cup water
- A pinch of crushed eggshell (for calcium)

**Preparation Time:**

- **Prep Time**: 10 minutes
- **Cook Time**: 4 hours on low
- **Total Time**: 4 hours 10 minutes
- **Difficulty Level**: Easy

**Instructions:**

1. **Prepare the Ingredients**:
    - Cube the turkey breast.
    - Rinse the brown rice.
    - Cook and mash the pumpkin.
    - Chop the carrots.
    - Measure out the peas.
2. **Combine in Slow Cooker**:
    - Place the turkey, brown rice, pumpkin, peas, and carrots in the slow cooker.
    - Add 1 cup of water to ensure there is enough moisture.
    - Drizzle with olive oil or fish oil (optional).

3. **Cook**:
   - Set the slow cooker to low and cook for 4 hours or until the turkey is fully cooked and the vegetables are tender.
4. **Cool and Serve**:
   - Allow the mixture to cool to a safe temperature before serving.
   - Portion according to your dog's size and daily caloric needs.

## Nutritional Information (per serving):

| Nutrient | Quantity (per cup) | Daily Value (%) |
|---|---|---|
| Calories | 157 kcal | - |
| Protein | 0.63 oz (18.24 g) | 47.72% |
| Fat | 0.03 oz (1.31 g) | 8.37% |
| Carbohydrates | 0.77 oz (22.67 g) | 43.91% |
| Fiber | 0.07 oz (2.31 g) | 2.31% |

## Suggested Portions (Daily):

| Dog Size (lbs) | Low Activity | Moderate Activity | High Activity |
|---|---|---|---|
| 5 | 1/2 cup | 3/4 cup | 1 cup |
| 10 | 1 cup | 1 1/2 cups | 2 cups |
| 20 | 2 cups | 2 1/2 cups | 3 cups |
| 30 | 2 1/2 cups | 3 1/2 cups | 4 cups |
| 40 | 3 cups | 4 cups | 5 cups |
| 50 | 3 1/2 cups | 4 1/2 cups | 5 1/2 cups |
| 60 | 4 cups | 5 cups | 6 cups |
| 70 | 4 1/2 cups | 5 1/2 cups | 6 1/2 cups |
| 80 | 5 cups | 6 cups | 7 cups |
| 90 | 5 1/2 cups | 6 1/2 cups | 7 1/2 cups |
| 100 | 6 cups | 7 cups | 8 cups |

# Beef Recipes

## Recipe 1: Beef, Sweet Potato, and Blueberry Delight

**Ingredients (for 1 cup):**

- 1.6 oz lean beef, cubed
- 1/4 cup sweet potatoes, diced
- 1/4 cup green beans, chopped
- 1/4 cup blueberries
- 1/4 cup spinach, chopped
- 1/2 tsp olive oil or fish oil (optional)
- 1 cup water
- A pinch of crushed eggshell (for calcium)

**Preparation Time:**

- **Prep Time**: 10 minutes
- **Cook Time**: 4 hours on low
- **Total Time**: 4 hours 10 minutes
- **Difficulty Level**: Easy

**Instructions:**

1. **Prepare the Ingredients**:
    - Cube the beef.
    - Dice the sweet potatoes.
    - Chop the green beans and spinach.
    - Measure out the blueberries.
2. **Combine in Slow Cooker**:
    - Place the beef, sweet potatoes, green beans, blueberries, and spinach in the slow cooker.
    - Add 1 cup of water to ensure there is enough moisture.
    - Drizzle with olive oil or fish oil (optional).
3. **Cook**:
    - Set the slow cooker to low and cook for 4 hours or until the beef is fully cooked and the vegetables are tender.
4. **Cool and Serve**:
    - Allow the mixture to cool to a safe temperature before serving.
    - Portion according to your dog's size and daily caloric needs.

### Nutritional Information (per serving):

| Nutrient | Quantity (per cup) | Daily Value (%) |
|---|---|---|
| Calories | 181 kcal | - |
| Protein | 0.60 oz (17.99 g) | 37.92% |
| Fat | 0.25 oz (5.14 g) | 26.27% |
| Carbohydrates | 0.75 oz (20.45 g) | 35.82% |
| Fiber | 0.04 oz (1.31 g) | 2.53% |

## Suggested Portions (Daily):

| Dog Size (lbs) | Low Activity | Moderate Activity | High Activity |
|---|---|---|---|
| 5 | 1/2 cup | 3/4 cup | 1 cup |
| 10 | 1 cup | 1 1/2 cups | 2 cups |
| 20 | 2 cups | 2 1/2 cups | 3 cups |
| 30 | 2 1/2 cups | 3 1/2 cups | 4 cups |
| 40 | 3 cups | 4 cups | 5 cups |
| 50 | 3 1/2 cups | 4 1/2 cups | 5 1/2 cups |
| 60 | 4 cups | 5 cups | 6 cups |
| 70 | 4 1/2 cups | 5 1/2 cups | 6 1/2 cups |
| 80 | 5 cups | 6 cups | 7 cups |
| 90 | 5 1/2 cups | 6 1/2 cups | 7 1/2 cups |
| 100 | 6 cups | 7 cups | 8 cups |

## Recipe 2: Beef, Rice, and Veggie Medley

**Ingredients (for 1 cup):**

- 1.2 oz lean beef, cubed (ridotta per diminuire il contenuto di grassi)
- 2 tbsp brown rice, rinsed
- 1/4 cup carrots, chopped
- 1/4 cup spinach, chopped
- 1/4 cup green beans, chopped
- 1/4 cup peas
- 1/4 cup pumpkin, cooked and mashed (aggiunta per bilanciare i nutrienti)
- 1/4 tsp flaxseed oil or fish oil (ridotta per diminuire il contenuto di grassi)
- 1 cup water
- A pinch of crushed eggshell (for calcium)

**Preparation Time:**

- **Prep Time**: 10 minutes
- **Cook Time**: 4 hours on low
- **Total Time**: 4 hours 10 minutes
- **Difficulty Level**: Easy

**Instructions:**

1. **Prepare the Ingredients**:
   - Cube the beef.
   - Rinse the brown rice.
   - Chop the carrots, spinach, green beans, and measure out the peas and pumpkin.
2. **Combine in Slow Cooker**:
   - Place the beef, brown rice, carrots, spinach, green beans, peas, and pumpkin in the slow cooker.
   - Add 1 cup of water to ensure there is enough moisture.
   - Drizzle with flaxseed oil or fish oil (optional).
3. **Cook**:

- Set the slow cooker to low and cook for 4 hours or until the beef is fully cooked and the vegetables are tender.
4. **Cool and Serve**:
    - Allow the mixture to cool to a safe temperature before serving.
    - Portion according to your dog's size and daily caloric needs.

## Nutritional Information (per serving):

| Nutrient | Quantity (per cup) | Daily Value (%) |
|---|---|---|
| Calories | 172 kcal | - |
| Protein | 0.56 oz (15.85 g) | 36.72% |
| Fat | 0.15 oz (4.25 g) | 13.05% |
| Carbohydrates | 0.74 oz (21.00 g) | 47.67% |
| Fiber | 0.07 oz (2.10 g) | 2.10% |

## Suggested Portions (Daily):

| Dog Size (lbs) | Low Activity | Moderate Activity | High Activity |
|---|---|---|---|
| 5 | 1/2 cup | 3/4 cup | 1 cup |
| 10 | 1 cup | 1 1/2 cups | 2 cups |
| 20 | 2 cups | 2 1/2 cups | 3 cups |
| 30 | 2 1/2 cups | 3 1/2 cups | 4 cups |
| 40 | 3 cups | 4 cups | 5 cups |
| 50 | 3 1/2 cups | 4 1/2 cups | 5 1/2 cups |
| 60 | 4 cups | 5 cups | 6 cups |
| 70 | 4 1/2 cups | 5 1/2 cups | 6 1/2 cups |
| 80 | 5 cups | 6 cups | 7 cups |
| 90 | 5 1/2 cups | 6 1/2 cups | 7 1/2 cups |
| 100 | 6 cups | 7 cups | 8 cups |

## Recipe 3: Beef, Quinoa, and Apple Delight

**Ingredients (for 1 cup):**

- 1 oz lean beef, cubed
- 3 tbsp quinoa, rinsed
- 1/4 cup broccoli, chopped
- 1/4 cup apples, chopped
- 1/4 cup carrots, chopped
- 1/4 cup peas
- 1/4 tsp olive oil or fish oil (optional)
- 1 cup water
- A pinch of crushed eggshell (for calcium)

**Preparation Time:**

- **Prep Time**: 10 minutes
- **Cook Time**: 4 hours on low

- **Total Time**: 4 hours 10 minutes
- **Difficulty Level**: Easy

**Instructions:**

1. **Prepare the Ingredients**:
   - Cube the beef.
   - Rinse the quinoa.
   - Chop the broccoli, apples, and carrots.
2. **Combine in Slow Cooker**:
   - Place the beef, quinoa, broccoli, apples, carrots, and peas in the slow cooker.
   - Add 1 cup of water to ensure there is enough moisture.
   - Drizzle with olive oil or fish oil (optional).
3. **Cook**:
   - Set the slow cooker to low and cook for 4 hours or until the beef is fully cooked and the vegetables are tender.
4. **Cool and Serve**:
   - Allow the mixture to cool to a safe temperature before serving.
   - Portion according to your dog's size and daily caloric needs.

## Nutritional Information (per serving):

| Nutrient | Quantity (per cup) | Daily Value (%) |
|---|---|---|
| Calories | 160 kcal | - |
| Protein | 0.35 oz (9.92 g) | 31.0% |
| Fat | 0.05 oz (1.41 g) | 10.3% |
| Carbohydrates | 0.85 oz (24.03 g) | 58.7% |
| Fiber | 0.07 oz (2.10 g) | 2.10% |

## Suggested Portions (Daily):

| Dog Size (lbs) | Low Activity | Moderate Activity | High Activity |
|---|---|---|---|
| 5 | 1/2 cup | 3/4 cup | 1 cup |
| 10 | 1 cup | 1 1/2 cups | 2 cups |
| 20 | 2 cups | 2 1/2 cups | 3 cups |
| 30 | 2 1/2 cups | 3 1/2 cups | 4 cups |
| 40 | 3 cups | 4 cups | 5 cups |
| 50 | 3 1/2 cups | 4 1/2 cups | 5 1/2 cups |
| 60 | 4 cups | 5 cups | 6 cups |
| 70 | 4 1/2 cups | 5 1/2 cups | 6 1/2 cups |
| 80 | 5 cups | 6 cups | 7 cups |
| 90 | 5 1/2 cups | 6 1/2 cups | 7 1/2 cups |
| 100 | 6 cups | 7 cups | 8 cups |

# Recipe 4: Beef, Rice, and Veggie Bowl

**Ingredients (for 1 cup):**

- 1 oz lean beef, cubed
- 2 tbsp brown rice, rinsed
- 1/4 cup green peas
- 1/4 cup sweet potatoes, diced
- 1/4 cup zucchini, chopped
- 1/4 tsp olive oil or fish oil (optional)
- 1 cup water
- A pinch of crushed eggshell (for calcium)

**Preparation Time:**

- **Prep Time**: 10 minutes
- **Cook Time**: 4 hours on low
- **Total Time**: 4 hours 10 minutes
- **Difficulty Level**: Easy

**Instructions:**

1. **Prepare the Ingredients**:
    - Cube the beef.
    - Rinse the brown rice.
    - Dice the sweet potatoes.
    - Chop the zucchini and measure out the green peas.
2. **Combine in Slow Cooker**:
    - Place the beef, brown rice, green peas, sweet potatoes, and zucchini in the slow cooker.
    - Add 1 cup of water to ensure there is enough moisture.
    - Drizzle with olive oil or fish oil (optional).
3. **Cook**:
    - Set the slow cooker to low and cook for 4 hours or until the beef is fully cooked and the vegetables are tender.
4. **Cool and Serve**:
    - Allow the mixture to cool to a safe temperature before serving.
    - Portion according to your dog's size and daily caloric needs.

## Nutritional Information (per serving):

| Nutrient | Quantity (per cup) | Daily Value (%) |
|---|---|---|
| Calories | 180 kcal | - |
| Protein | 0.30 oz (8.96 g) | 29.72% |
| Fat | 0.05 oz (1.39 g) | 15.49% |
| Carbohydrates | 0.96 oz (26.54 g) | 54.78% |
| Fiber | 0.07 oz (2.13 g) | 2.13% |

## Suggested Portions (Daily):

| Dog Size (lbs) | Low Activity | Moderate Activity | High Activity |
|---|---|---|---|
| 5 | 1/2 cup | 3/4 cup | 1 cup |
| 10 | 1 cup | 1 1/2 cups | 2 cups |
| 20 | 2 cups | 2 1/2 cups | 3 cups |
| 30 | 2 1/2 cups | 3 1/2 cups | 4 cups |
| 40 | 3 cups | 4 cups | 5 cups |
| 50 | 3 1/2 cups | 4 1/2 cups | 5 1/2 cups |
| 60 | 4 cups | 5 cups | 6 cups |
| 70 | 4 1/2 cups | 5 1/2 cups | 6 1/2 cups |
| 80 | 5 cups | 6 cups | 7 cups |
| 90 | 5 1/2 cups | 6 1/2 cups | 7 1/2 cups |
| 100 | 6 cups | 7 cups | 8 cups |

## Recipe 5: Beef, Oats, and Veggie Delight

**Ingredients (for 1 cup):**

- 1 oz lean beef, cubed
- 3 tbsp oats, rinsed
- 1/4 cup spinach, chopped
- 1/4 cup carrots, chopped
- 1/4 cup pumpkin, cooked and mashed
- 1/4 cup peas
- 1/4 tsp olive oil or fish oil (optional)
- 1/4 cup brown rice, cooked
- 1 cup water
- A pinch of crushed eggshell (for calcium)

**Preparation Time:**

- **Prep Time**: 10 minutes
- **Cook Time**: 4 hours on low
- **Total Time**: 4 hours 10 minutes
- **Difficulty Level**: Easy

**Instructions:**

1. **Prepare the Ingredients**:
    - Cube the beef.
    - Rinse the oats.
    - Chop the spinach and carrots.
    - Cook and mash the pumpkin.
    - Measure out the peas and cook the brown rice.
2. **Combine in Slow Cooker**:
    - Place the beef, oats, spinach, carrots, pumpkin, peas, and brown rice in the slow cooker.
    - Add 1 cup of water to ensure there is enough moisture.
    - Drizzle with olive oil or fish oil (optional).

3. **Cook**:
   - Set the slow cooker to low and cook for 4 hours or until the beef is fully cooked and the vegetables are tender.
4. **Cool and Serve**:
   - Allow the mixture to cool to a safe temperature before serving.
   - Portion according to your dog's size and daily caloric needs.

## Nutritional Information (per serving):

| Nutrient | Quantity (per cup) | Daily Value (%) |
|---|---|---|
| Calories | 185 kcal | - |
| Protein | 0.35 oz (9.92 g) | 33.5% |
| Fat | 0.04 oz (1.12 g) | 10.5% |
| Carbohydrates | 0.85 oz (24.03 g) | 56.0% |
| Fiber | 0.05 oz (1.70 g) | 2.5% |

## Suggested Portions (Daily):

| Dog Size (lbs) | Low Activity | Moderate Activity | High Activity |
|---|---|---|---|
| 5 | 1 cup | 1 1/4 cups | 1 1/2 cups |
| 10 | 1 1/2 cups | 2 cups | 2 1/2 cups |
| 20 | 2 1/2 cups | 3 cups | 3 1/2 cups |
| 30 | 3 cups | 4 cups | 4 1/2 cups |
| 40 | 3 1/2 cups | 4 1/2 cups | 5 cups |
| 50 | 4 cups | 5 cups | 6 cups |
| 60 | 4 1/2 cups | 5 1/2 cups | 6 1/2 cups |
| 70 | 5 cups | 6 cups | 7 cups |
| 80 | 5 1/2 cups | 6 1/2 cups | 7 1/2 cups |
| 90 | 6 cups | 7 cups | 8 cups |
| 100 | 6 1/2 cups | 7 1/2 cups | 8 1/2 cups |

# Lamb Recipes

## Recipe 1: Lamb, Rice, and Veggie Feast

**Ingredients (for 1 cup):**

- 1 oz lean lamb, cubed
- 2 tbsp brown rice, rinsed
- 1/4 cup carrots, chopped
- 1/4 cup spinach, chopped
- 1/4 cup sweet potatoes, diced
- 1/4 cup peas
- 1/8 tsp olive oil or fish oil (optional)
- 1 cup water
- A pinch of crushed eggshell (for calcium)

**Preparation Time:**

- **Prep Time**: 10 minutes
- **Cook Time**: 4 hours on low
- **Total Time**: 4 hours 10 minutes
- **Difficulty Level**: Easy

**Instructions:**

1. **Prepare the Ingredients**:
    - Cube the lamb.
    - Rinse the brown rice.
    - Chop the carrots, spinach, and sweet potatoes.
    - Measure out the peas.
2. **Combine in Slow Cooker**:
    - Place the lamb, brown rice, carrots, spinach, sweet potatoes, and peas in the slow cooker.
    - Add 1 cup of water to ensure there is enough moisture.
    - Drizzle with olive oil or fish oil (optional).
3. **Cook**:
    - Set the slow cooker to low and cook for 4 hours or until the lamb is fully cooked and the vegetables are tender.
4. **Cool and Serve**:
    - Allow the mixture to cool to a safe temperature before serving.
    - Portion according to your dog's size and daily caloric needs.

## Nutritional Information (per serving):

| Nutrient | Quantity (per cup) | Daily Value (%) |
|---|---|---|
| Calories | 180 kcal | - |
| Protein | 0.35 oz (9.9 g) | 30.0% |
| Fat | 0.02 oz (0.9 g) | 15.0% |
| Carbohydrates | 0.85 oz (24 g) | 50.0% |
| Fiber | 0.04 oz (1.2 g) | 2.0% |

## Suggested Portions (Daily):

| Dog Size (lbs) | Low Activity | Moderate Activity | High Activity |
|---|---|---|---|
| 5 | 1 cup | 1 1/4 cups | 1 1/2 cups |
| 10 | 1 1/2 cups | 2 cups | 2 1/2 cups |
| 20 | 2 1/2 cups | 3 cups | 3 1/2 cups |
| 30 | 3 cups | 4 cups | 4 1/2 cups |
| 40 | 3 1/2 cups | 4 1/2 cups | 5 cups |
| 50 | 4 cups | 5 cups | 6 cups |
| 60 | 4 1/2 cups | 5 1/2 cups | 6 1/2 cups |
| 70 | 5 cups | 6 cups | 7 cups |
| 80 | 5 1/2 cups | 6 1/2 cups | 7 1/2 cups |
| 90 | 6 cups | 7 cups | 8 cups |
| 100 | 6 1/2 cups | 7 1/2 cups | 8 1/2 cups |

## Recipe 2: Lamb Harvest Feast

**Ingredients (for 1 cup):**

- 1.2 oz lean lamb, cubed
- 2 tbsp quinoa, rinsed
- 1/4 cup broccoli, chopped
- 1/4 cup carrots, chopped
- 1/4 cup pumpkin, cooked and mashed
- 1/4 cup peas
- 1/4 tsp olive oil or fish oil (optional)
- 1 cup water
- A pinch of crushed eggshell (for calcium)

**Preparation Time:**

- **Prep Time**: 10 minutes
- **Cook Time**: 4 hours on low
- **Total Time**: 4 hours 10 minutes
- **Difficulty Level**: Easy

**Instructions:**

1. **Prepare the Ingredients**:
    - Cube the lamb.
    - Rinse the quinoa.
    - Chop the broccoli and carrots.
    - Cook and mash the pumpkin.
    - Measure out the peas.
2. **Combine in Slow Cooker**:
    - Place the lamb, quinoa, broccoli, carrots, pumpkin, and peas in the slow cooker.
    - Add 1 cup of water to ensure there is enough moisture.
    - Drizzle with olive oil or fish oil (optional).

3. **Cook**:
   - Set the slow cooker to low and cook for 4 hours or until the lamb is fully cooked and the vegetables are tender.
4. **Cool and Serve**:
   - Allow the mixture to cool to a safe temperature before serving.
   - Portion according to your dog's size and daily caloric needs.

## Nutritional Information (per serving):

| Nutrient | Quantity (per cup) | Daily Value (%) |
|---|---|---|
| Calories | 180 kcal | - |
| Protein | 0.40 oz (11.2 g) | 33.3% |
| Fat | 0.02 oz (0.8 g) | 15.0% |
| Carbohydrates | 0.85 oz (24.5 g) | 48.0% |
| Fiber | 0.04 oz (1.0 g) | 3.0% |

## Suggested Portions (Daily):

| Dog Size (lbs) | Low Activity | Moderate Activity | High Activity |
|---|---|---|---|
| 5 | 1 cup | 1 1/4 cups | 1 1/2 cups |
| 10 | 1 1/2 cups | 2 cups | 2 1/2 cups |
| 20 | 2 1/2 cups | 3 cups | 3 1/2 cups |
| 30 | 3 cups | 4 cups | 4 1/2 cups |
| 40 | 3 1/2 cups | 4 1/2 cups | 5 cups |
| 50 | 4 cups | 5 cups | 6 cups |
| 60 | 4 1/2 cups | 5 1/2 cups | 6 1/2 cups |
| 70 | 5 cups | 6 cups | 7 cups |
| 80 | 5 1/2 cups | 6 1/2 cups | 7 1/2 cups |
| 90 | 6 cups | 7 cups | 8 cups |
| 100 | 6 1/2 cups | 7 1/2 cups | 8 1/2 cups |

## Recipe 3: Lamb & Veggie Power Bowl

**Ingredients (for 1 cup):**

- 1 oz lean lamb, cubed
- 2 tbsp brown rice, rinsed
- 1/4 cup carrots, chopped
- 1/4 cup spinach, chopped
- 1/4 cup sweet potatoes, diced
- 1/4 cup green peas
- 1/8 tsp olive oil or fish oil (optional)
- 1 cup water
- A pinch of crushed eggshell (for calcium)

**Preparation Time:**

- **Prep Time**: 10 minutes

- **Cook Time**: 4 hours on low
- **Total Time**: 4 hours 10 minutes
- **Difficulty Level**: Easy

**Instructions:**

1. **Prepare the Ingredients**:
    - Cube the lamb.
    - Rinse the brown rice.
    - Chop the carrots, spinach, and sweet potatoes.
    - Measure out the green peas.
2. **Combine in Slow Cooker**:
    - Place the lamb, brown rice, carrots, spinach, sweet potatoes, and green peas in the slow cooker.
    - Add 1 cup of water to ensure there is enough moisture.
    - Drizzle with olive oil or fish oil (optional).
3. **Cook**:
    - Set the slow cooker to low and cook for 4 hours or until the lamb is fully cooked and the vegetables are tender.
4. **Cool and Serve**:
    - Allow the mixture to cool to a safe temperature before serving.
    - Portion according to your dog's size and daily caloric needs.

## Nutritional Information (per serving):

| Nutrient | Quantity (per cup) | Daily Value (%) |
|---|---|---|
| Calories | 192 kcal | - |
| Protein | 0.40 oz (11.2 g) | 28.0% |
| Fat | 0.02 oz (0.9 g) | 17.8% |
| Carbohydrates | 0.85 oz (24.5 g) | 54.2% |
| Fiber | 0.04 oz (1.2 g) | 2.3% |

## Suggested Portions (Daily):

| Dog Size (lbs) | Low Activity | Moderate Activity | High Activity |
|---|---|---|---|
| 5 | 1 cup | 1 1/4 cups | 1 1/2 cups |
| 10 | 1 1/2 cups | 2 cups | 2 1/2 cups |
| 20 | 2 1/2 cups | 3 cups | 3 1/2 cups |
| 30 | 3 cups | 4 cups | 4 1/2 cups |
| 40 | 3 1/2 cups | 4 1/2 cups | 5 cups |
| 50 | 4 cups | 5 cups | 6 cups |
| 60 | 4 1/2 cups | 5 1/2 cups | 6 1/2 cups |
| 70 | 5 cups | 6 cups | 7 cups |
| 80 | 5 1/2 cups | 6 1/2 cups | 7 1/2 cups |
| 90 | 6 cups | 7 cups | 8 cups |
| 100 | 6 1/2 cups | 7 1/2 cups | 8 1/2 cups |

# Recipe 4: Lamb and Harvest Veggie Feast

**Ingredients (for 1 cup):**

- 1 oz lean lamb, cubed
- 1 tbsp brown rice, rinsed
- 1/4 cup carrots, chopped
- 1/4 cup spinach, chopped
- 1/4 cup sweet potatoes, diced
- 1/4 cup green peas
- 1/8 tsp olive oil or fish oil (optional)
- 1 cup water
- A pinch of crushed eggshell (for calcium)

**Preparation Time:**

- **Prep Time**: 10 minutes
- **Cook Time**: 4 hours on low
- **Total Time**: 4 hours 10 minutes
- **Difficulty Level**: Easy

**Instructions:**

1. **Prepare the Ingredients**:
    - Cube the lamb.
    - Rinse the brown rice.
    - Chop the carrots, spinach, and sweet potatoes.
    - Measure out the green peas.
2. **Combine in Slow Cooker**:
    - Place the lamb, brown rice, carrots, spinach, sweet potatoes, and green peas in the slow cooker.
    - Add 1 cup of water to ensure there is enough moisture.
    - Drizzle with olive oil or fish oil (optional).
3. **Cook**:
    - Set the slow cooker to low and cook for 4 hours or until the lamb is fully cooked and the vegetables are tender.
4. **Cool and Serve**:
    - Allow the mixture to cool to a safe temperature before serving.
    - Portion according to your dog's size and daily caloric needs.

## Nutritional Information (per serving):

| Nutrient | Quantity (per cup) | Daily Value (%) |
| --- | --- | --- |
| Calories | 160 kcal | - |
| Protein | 0.33 oz (9.3 g) | 28.0% |
| Fat | 0.02 oz (0.7 g) | 15.0% |
| Carbohydrates | 0.85 oz (24.0 g) | 55.0% |
| Fiber | 0.04 oz (1.3 g) | 2.5% |

## Suggested Portions (Daily):

| Dog Size (lbs) | Low Activity | Moderate Activity | High Activity |
|---|---|---|---|
| 5 | 1 cup | 1 1/4 cups | 1 1/2 cups |
| 10 | 1 1/2 cups | 2 cups | 2 1/2 cups |
| 20 | 2 1/2 cups | 3 cups | 3 1/2 cups |
| 30 | 3 cups | 4 cups | 4 1/2 cups |
| 40 | 3 1/2 cups | 4 1/2 cups | 5 cups |
| 50 | 4 cups | 5 cups | 6 cups |
| 60 | 4 1/2 cups | 5 1/2 cups | 6 1/2 cups |
| 70 | 5 cups | 6 cups | 7 cups |
| 80 | 5 1/2 cups | 6 1/2 cups | 7 1/2 cups |
| 90 | 6 cups | 7 cups | 8 cups |
| 100 | 6 1/2 cups | 7 1/2 cups | 8 1/2 cups |

## Recipe 5: Lamb and Autumn Harvest Medley

**Ingredients (for 1 cup):**

- 1 oz lean lamb, cubed
- 1 tbsp quinoa, rinsed
- 1/4 cup zucchini, chopped
- 1/4 cup butternut squash, diced
- 1/4 cup green beans, chopped
- 1/4 cup apples, chopped
- 1/8 tsp olive oil or fish oil (optional)
- 1 cup water
- A pinch of crushed eggshell (for calcium)

**Preparation Time:**

- **Prep Time**: 10 minutes
- **Cook Time**: 4 hours on low
- **Total Time**: 4 hours 10 minutes
- **Difficulty Level**: Easy

**Instructions:**

1. **Prepare the Ingredients**:
   - Cube the lamb.
   - Rinse the quinoa.
   - Chop the zucchini, butternut squash, green beans, and apples.
2. **Combine in Slow Cooker**:
   - Place the lamb, quinoa, zucchini, butternut squash, green beans, and apples in the slow cooker.
   - Add 1 cup of water to ensure there is enough moisture.
   - Drizzle with olive oil or fish oil (optional).
3. **Cook**:

- Set the slow cooker to low and cook for 4 hours or until the lamb is fully cooked and the vegetables are tender.
4. **Cool and Serve**:
    - Allow the mixture to cool to a safe temperature before serving.
    - Portion according to your dog's size and daily caloric needs.

## Nutritional Information (per serving):

| Nutrient | Quantity (per cup) | Daily Value (%) |
|---|---|---|
| Calories | 160 kcal | - |
| Protein | 0.32 oz (9.1 g) | 30.0% |
| Fat | 0.02 oz (0.7 g) | 15.0% |
| Carbohydrates | 0.85 oz (24.0 g) | 55.0% |
| Fiber | 0.04 oz (1.3 g) | 2.5% |

## Suggested Portions (Daily):

| Dog Size (lbs) | Low Activity | Moderate Activity | High Activity |
|---|---|---|---|
| 5 | 1 cup | 1 1/4 cups | 1 1/2 cups |
| 10 | 1 1/2 cups | 2 cups | 2 1/2 cups |
| 20 | 2 1/2 cups | 3 cups | 3 1/2 cups |
| 30 | 3 cups | 4 cups | 4 1/2 cups |
| 40 | 3 1/2 cups | 4 1/2 cups | 5 cups |
| 50 | 4 cups | 5 cups | 6 cups |
| 60 | 4 1/2 cups | 5 1/2 cups | 6 1/2 cups |
| 70 | 5 cups | 6 cups | 7 cups |
| 80 | 5 1/2 cups | 6 1/2 cups | 7 1/2 cups |
| 90 | 6 cups | 7 cups | 8 cups |
| 100 | 6 1/2 cups | 7 1/2 cups | 8 1/2 cups |

# Pork Recipes

## Recipe 1: Pork and Garden Delight

**Ingredients (for 1 cup):**

- 0.8 oz lean pork, cubed
- 2 tbsp brown rice, rinsed
- 1/4 cup carrots, chopped
- 1/4 cup spinach, chopped
- 1/4 cup sweet potatoes, diced
- 1/4 cup green peas
- 1/8 tsp olive oil or fish oil (optional)
- 1 cup water
- A pinch of crushed eggshell (for calcium)

**Preparation Time:**

- **Prep Time**: 10 minutes
- **Cook Time**: 4 hours on low
- **Total Time**: 4 hours 10 minutes
- **Difficulty Level**: Easy

**Instructions:**

1. **Prepare the Ingredients**:
   - Cube the pork.
   - Rinse the brown rice.
   - Chop the carrots, spinach, and sweet potatoes.
   - Measure out the green peas.
2. **Combine in Slow Cooker**:
   - Place the pork, brown rice, carrots, spinach, sweet potatoes, and green peas in the slow cooker.
   - Add 1 cup of water to ensure there is enough moisture.
   - Drizzle with olive oil or fish oil (optional).
3. **Cook**:
   - Set the slow cooker to low and cook for 4 hours or until the pork is fully cooked and the vegetables are tender.
4. **Cool and Serve**:
   - Allow the mixture to cool to a safe temperature before serving.
   - Portion according to your dog's size and daily caloric needs.

## Nutritional Information (per serving):

| Nutrient | Quantity (per cup) | Daily Value (%) |
| --- | --- | --- |
| Calories | 160 kcal | - |
| Protein | 0.31 oz (8.4 g) | 31.0% |
| Fat | 0.02 oz (0.8 g) | 15.0% |
| Carbohydrates | 0.87 oz (24.0 g) | 55.0% |
| Fiber | 0.04 oz (1.3 g) | 2.5% |

## Suggested Portions (Daily):

| Dog Size (lbs) | Low Activity | Moderate Activity | High Activity |
|---|---|---|---|
| 5 | 1 cup | 1 1/4 cups | 1 1/2 cups |
| 10 | 1 1/2 cups | 2 cups | 2 1/2 cups |
| 20 | 2 1/2 cups | 3 cups | 3 1/2 cups |
| 30 | 3 cups | 4 cups | 4 1/2 cups |
| 40 | 3 1/2 cups | 4 1/2 cups | 5 cups |
| 50 | 4 cups | 5 cups | 6 cups |
| 60 | 4 1/2 cups | 5 1/2 cups | 6 1/2 cups |
| 70 | 5 cups | 6 cups | 7 cups |
| 80 | 5 1/2 cups | 6 1/2 cups | 7 1/2 cups |
| 90 | 6 cups | 7 cups | 8 cups |
| 100 | 6 1/2 cups | 7 1/2 cups | 8 1/2 cups |

## Recipe 2: Pork and Autumn Veggie Medley

**Ingredients (for 1 cup):**

- 1.2 oz lean pork, cubed
- 2 tbsp quinoa, rinsed
- 1/4 cup broccoli, chopped
- 1/4 cup carrots, chopped
- 1/4 cup pumpkin, cooked and mashed
- 1/4 cup peas
- 1/8 tsp olive oil or fish oil (optional)
- 1 cup water
- A pinch of crushed eggshell (for calcium)

**Preparation Time:**

- **Prep Time**: 10 minutes
- **Cook Time**: 4 hours on low
- **Total Time**: 4 hours 10 minutes
- **Difficulty Level**: Easy

**Instructions:**

1. **Prepare the Ingredients**:
    - Cube the pork.
    - Rinse the quinoa.
    - Chop the broccoli and carrots.
    - Cook and mash the pumpkin.
    - Measure out the peas.
2. **Combine in Slow Cooker**:
    - Place the pork, quinoa, broccoli, carrots, pumpkin, and peas in the slow cooker.
    - Add 1 cup of water to ensure there is enough moisture.
    - Drizzle with olive oil or fish oil (optional).

3. **Cook**:
   - Set the slow cooker to low and cook for 4 hours or until the pork is fully cooked and the vegetables are tender.
4. **Cool and Serve**:
   - Allow the mixture to cool to a safe temperature before serving.
   - Portion according to your dog's size and daily caloric needs.

## Nutritional Information (per serving):

| Nutrient | Quantity (per cup) | Daily Value (%) |
|---|---|---|
| Calories | 160 kcal | - |
| Protein | 0.37 oz (10.5 g) | 33.0% |
| Fat | 0.02 oz (0.9 g) | 15.0% |
| Carbohydrates | 0.90 oz (25.5 g) | 50.0% |
| Fiber | 0.04 oz (1.3 g) | 2.0% |

## Suggested Portions (Daily):

| Dog Size (lbs) | Low Activity | Moderate Activity | High Activity |
|---|---|---|---|
| 5 | 1 cup | 1 1/4 cups | 1 1/2 cups |
| 10 | 1 1/2 cups | 2 cups | 2 1/2 cups |
| 20 | 2 1/2 cups | 3 cups | 3 1/2 cups |
| 30 | 3 cups | 4 cups | 4 1/2 cups |
| 40 | 3 1/2 cups | 4 1/2 cups | 5 cups |
| 50 | 4 cups | 5 cups | 6 cups |
| 60 | 4 1/2 cups | 5 1/2 cups | 6 1/2 cups |
| 70 | 5 cups | 6 cups | 7 cups |
| 80 | 5 1/2 cups | 6 1/2 cups | 7 1/2 cups |
| 90 | 6 cups | 7 cups | 8 cups |
| 100 | 6 1/2 cups | 7 1/2 cups | 8 1/2 cups |

## Recipe 3: Pork and Winter Wonderland Feast

**Ingredients (for 1 cup):**

- 1.2 oz lean pork, cubed
- 2 tbsp brown rice, rinsed
- 1/4 cup zucchini, chopped
- 1/4 cup butternut squash, diced
- 1/4 cup green beans, chopped
- 1/4 cup apples, chopped
- 1/4 tsp olive oil or fish oil (optional)
- 1 cup water
- A pinch of crushed eggshell (for calcium)

**Preparation Time:**

- **Prep Time**: 10 minutes

- **Cook Time**: 4 hours on low
- **Total Time**: 4 hours 10 minutes
- **Difficulty Level**: Easy

**Instructions:**

1. **Prepare the Ingredients**:
    - Cube the pork.
    - Rinse the brown rice.
    - Chop the zucchini, butternut squash, green beans, and apples.
2. **Combine in Slow Cooker**:
    - Place the pork, brown rice, zucchini, butternut squash, green beans, and apples in the slow cooker.
    - Add 1 cup of water to ensure there is enough moisture.
    - Drizzle with olive oil or fish oil (optional).
3. **Cook**:
    - Set the slow cooker to low and cook for 4 hours or until the pork is fully cooked and the vegetables are tender.
4. **Cool and Serve**:
    - Allow the mixture to cool to a safe temperature before serving.
    - Portion according to your dog's size and daily caloric needs.

## Nutritional Information (per serving):

| Nutrient | Quantity (per cup) | Daily Value (%) |
|---|---|---|
| Calories | 160 kcal | - |
| Protein | 0.32 oz (9.1 g) | 29.4% |
| Fat | 0.02 oz (0.7 g) | 14.9% |
| Carbohydrates | 0.90 oz (25.5 g) | 55.6% |
| Fiber | 0.04 oz (1.4 g) | 2.5% |

## Suggested Portions (Daily):

| Dog Size (lbs) | Low Activity | Moderate Activity | High Activity |
|---|---|---|---|
| 5 | 1 cup | 1 1/4 cups | 1 1/2 cups |
| 10 | 1 1/2 cups | 2 cups | 2 1/2 cups |
| 20 | 2 1/2 cups | 3 cups | 3 1/2 cups |
| 30 | 3 cups | 4 cups | 4 1/2 cups |
| 40 | 3 1/2 cups | 4 1/2 cups | 5 cups |
| 50 | 4 cups | 5 cups | 6 cups |
| 60 | 4 1/2 cups | 5 1/2 cups | 6 1/2 cups |
| 70 | 5 cups | 6 cups | 7 cups |
| 80 | 5 1/2 cups | 6 1/2 cups | 7 1/2 cups |
| 90 | 6 cups | 7 cups | 8 cups |
| 100 | 6 1/2 cups | 7 1/2 cups | 8 1/2 cups |

## Recipe 4: Pork and Summer Harvest Delight

**Ingredients (for 1 cup):**

- 1 oz lean pork, cubed
- 1 tbsp quinoa, rinsed
- 1/4 cup carrots, chopped
- 1/4 cup spinach, chopped
- 1/4 cup sweet potatoes, diced
- 1/4 cup green peas
- 1/8 tsp olive oil or fish oil (optional)
- 1 cup water
- A pinch of crushed eggshell (for calcium)

**Preparation Time:**

- **Prep Time**: 10 minutes
- **Cook Time**: 4 hours on low
- **Total Time**: 4 hours 10 minutes
- **Difficulty Level**: Easy

**Instructions:**

1. **Prepare the Ingredients**:
    - Cube the pork.
    - Rinse the quinoa.
    - Chop the carrots, spinach, and sweet potatoes.
    - Measure out the green peas.
2. **Combine in Slow Cooker**:
    - Place the pork, quinoa, carrots, spinach, sweet potatoes, and green peas in the slow cooker.
    - Add 1 cup of water to ensure there is enough moisture.
    - Drizzle with olive oil or fish oil (optional).
3. **Cook**:
    - Set the slow cooker to low and cook for 4 hours or until the pork is fully cooked and the vegetables are tender.
4. **Cool and Serve**:
    - Allow the mixture to cool to a safe temperature before serving.
    - Portion according to your dog's size and daily caloric needs.

## Nutritional Information (per serving):

| Nutrient | Quantity (per cup) | Daily Value (%) |
|---|---|---|
| Calories | 165 kcal | - |
| Protein | 0.30 oz (8.5 g) | 30.0% |
| Fat | 0.02 oz (0.7 g) | 15.0% |
| Carbohydrates | 0.88 oz (25.0 g) | 50.0% |
| Fiber | 0.03 oz (1.1 g) | 2.5% |

## Suggested Portions (Daily):

| Dog Size (lbs) | Low Activity | Moderate Activity | High Activity |
|---|---|---|---|
| 5 | 1 cup | 1 1/4 cups | 1 1/2 cups |
| 10 | 1 1/2 cups | 2 cups | 2 1/2 cups |
| 20 | 2 1/2 cups | 3 cups | 3 1/2 cups |
| 30 | 3 cups | 4 cups | 4 1/2 cups |
| 40 | 3 1/2 cups | 4 1/2 cups | 5 cups |
| 50 | 4 cups | 5 cups | 6 cups |
| 60 | 4 1/2 cups | 5 1/2 cups | 6 1/2 cups |
| 70 | 5 cups | 6 cups | 7 cups |
| 80 | 5 1/2 cups | 6 1/2 cups | 7 1/2 cups |
| 90 | 6 cups | 7 cups | 8 cups |
| 100 | 6 1/2 cups | 7 1/2 cups | 8 1/2 cups |

## Recipe 5: Pork and Blueberry Picnic Bowl

**Ingredients (for 1 cup):**

- 1 oz lean pork, cubed
- 2 tbsp brown rice, rinsed
- 1/4 cup blueberries
- 1/3 cup broccoli, chopped
- 1/3 cup carrots, chopped
- 1/8 tsp olive oil or fish oil (optional)
- 1 cup water
- A pinch of crushed eggshell (for calcium)

**Preparation Time:**

- **Prep Time**: 10 minutes
- **Cook Time**: 4 hours on low
- **Total Time**: 4 hours 10 minutes
- **Difficulty Level**: Easy

**Instructions:**

1. **Prepare the Ingredients**:
    - Cube the pork.
    - Rinse the brown rice.
    - Measure out the blueberries.
    - Chop the broccoli and carrots.
2. **Combine in Slow Cooker**:
    - Place the pork, brown rice, blueberries, broccoli, and carrots in the slow cooker.
    - Add 1 cup of water to ensure there is enough moisture.
    - Drizzle with olive oil or fish oil (optional).

3. **Cook**:
    - Set the slow cooker to low and cook for 4 hours or until the pork is fully cooked and the vegetables are tender.
4. **Cool and Serve**:
    - Allow the mixture to cool to a safe temperature before serving.
    - Portion according to your dog's size and daily caloric needs.

## Nutritional Information (per serving):

| Nutrient | Quantity (per cup) | Daily Value (%) |
|---|---|---|
| Calories | 167 kcal | - |
| Protein | 0.31 oz (8.9 g) | 30.5% |
| Fat | 0.02 oz (0.7 g) | 14.9% |
| Carbohydrates | 0.86 oz (24.2 g) | 54.6% |
| Fiber | 0.04 oz (1.7 g) | 1.7% |

## Suggested Portions (Daily):

| Dog Size (lbs) | Low Activity | Moderate Activity | High Activity |
|---|---|---|---|
| 5 | 1 cup | 1 1/4 cups | 1 1/2 cups |
| 10 | 1 1/2 cups | 2 cups | 2 1/2 cups |
| 20 | 2 1/2 cups | 3 cups | 3 1/2 cups |
| 30 | 3 cups | 4 cups | 4 1/2 cups |
| 40 | 3 1/2 cups | 4 1/2 cups | 5 cups |
| 50 | 4 cups | 5 cups | 6 cups |
| 60 | 4 1/2 cups | 5 1/2 cups | 6 1/2 cups |
| 70 | 5 cups | 6 cups | 7 cups |
| 80 | 5 1/2 cups | 6 1/2 cups | 7 1/2 cups |
| 90 | 6 cups | 7 cups | 8 cups |
| 100 | 6 1/2 cups | 7 1/2 cups | 8 1/2 cups |

# Egg Recipes

## Recipe 1: Egg and Veggie Sunrise Delight

**Ingredients (for 1 cup):**

- 1 large egg (50g)
- 2 tbsp quinoa, cooked (30g)
- 1/4 cup spinach, chopped (30g)
- 1/4 cup sweet potatoes, diced (30g)
- 1/4 cup zucchini, chopped (30g)
- 1/4 cup carrots, chopped (30g)
- 1/2 tsp olive oil (2.5g)
- 1 cup water

**Preparation Time:**

- **Prep Time**: 10 minutes
- **Cook Time**: 4 hours
- **Total Time**: 4 hours 10 minutes
- **Difficulty Level**: Easy

**Instructions:**

1. **Prepare the Ingredients**:
    - Cook the quinoa according to package instructions.
    - Dice the sweet potatoes.
    - Chop the spinach, zucchini, and carrots.
    - Beat the egg lightly.
2. **Combine in the Slow Cooker**:
    - Place the sweet potatoes, zucchini, carrots, spinach, and cooked quinoa in the slow cooker.
    - Pour the beaten egg over the vegetable-quinoa mixture.
    - Add olive oil and water.
3. **Cook**:
    - Set the slow cooker to low and cook for 4 hours or until the vegetables are tender and the egg is fully cooked and mixed with the vegetables and quinoa.
4. **Cool and Serve**:
    - Allow the mixture to cool to a safe temperature before serving.
    - Portion according to your dog's size and daily caloric needs.

## Nutritional Information (per serving):

| Nutrient | Quantity (per cup) | Daily Value (%) |
|---|---|---|
| Calories | 162 kcal | - |
| Protein | 0.32 oz (9.0 g) | 32.0% |
| Fat | 0.03 oz (1.1 g) | 15.0% |
| Carbohydrates | 0.85 oz (24.1 g) | 52.0% |
| Fiber | 0.05 oz (1.6 g) | 2.5% |

## Suggested Portions (Daily):

| Dog Size (lbs) | Low Activity | Moderate Activity | High Activity |
|---|---|---|---|
| 5 | 1 cup | 1 1/4 cups | 1 1/2 cups |
| 10 | 1 1/2 cups | 2 cups | 2 1/2 cups |
| 20 | 2 1/2 cups | 3 cups | 3 1/2 cups |
| 30 | 3 cups | 4 cups | 4 1/2 cups |
| 40 | 3 1/2 cups | 4 1/2 cups | 5 cups |
| 50 | 4 cups | 5 cups | 6 cups |
| 60 | 4 1/2 cups | 5 1/2 cups | 6 1/2 cups |
| 70 | 5 cups | 6 cups | 7 cups |
| 80 | 5 1/2 cups | 6 1/2 cups | 7 1/2 cups |
| 90 | 6 cups | 7 cups | 8 cups |
| 100 | 6 1/2 cups | 7 1/2 cups | 8 1/2 cups |

## Recipe 2: Egg and Autumn Harvest Mix

**Ingredients (for 1 cup):**

- 1 large egg (50g)
- 2 tbsp brown rice, cooked (30g)
- 1/3 cup green beans, chopped (50g)
- 1/3 cup butternut squash, cooked and mashed (50g)
- 1/4 cup blueberries (30g)
- 1/16 tsp olive oil (0.3g)
- 1 cup water

**Preparation Time:**

- **Prep Time**: 10 minutes
- **Cook Time**: 4 hours
- **Total Time**: 4 hours 10 minutes
- **Difficulty Level**: Easy

**Instructions:**

1. **Prepare the Ingredients**:
    - Cook the brown rice according to package instructions.
    - Chop the green beans.
    - Cook and mash the butternut squash.

- o Measure out the blueberries.
- o Beat the egg lightly.
2. **Combine in the Slow Cooker**:
    - o Place the green beans, butternut squash, brown rice, and blueberries in the slow cooker.
    - o Pour the beaten egg over the vegetable-rice mixture.
    - o Add olive oil and water.
3. **Cook**:
    - o Set the slow cooker to low and cook for 4 hours or until the vegetables are tender and the egg is fully cooked and mixed with the vegetables and rice.
4. **Cool and Serve**:
    - o Allow the mixture to cool to a safe temperature before serving.
    - o Portion according to your dog's size and daily caloric needs.

## Nutritional Information (per serving):

| Nutrient | Quantity (per cup) | Daily Value (%) |
|---|---|---|
| Calories | 172 kcal | - |
| Protein | 0.31 oz (9.0 g) | 24.0% |
| Fat | 0.02 oz (0.7 g) | 17.0% |
| Carbohydrates | 0.86 oz (24.3 g) | 59.0% |
| Fiber | 0.05 oz (1.4 g) | 1.5% |

## Suggested Portions (Daily):

| Dog Size (lbs) | Low Activity | Moderate Activity | High Activity |
|---|---|---|---|
| 5 | 1 cup | 1 1/4 cups | 1 1/2 cups |
| 10 | 1 1/2 cups | 2 cups | 2 1/2 cups |
| 20 | 2 1/2 cups | 3 cups | 3 1/2 cups |
| 30 | 3 cups | 4 cups | 4 1/2 cups |
| 40 | 3 1/2 cups | 4 1/2 cups | 5 cups |
| 50 | 4 cups | 5 cups | 6 cups |
| 60 | 4 1/2 cups | 5 1/2 cups | 6 1/2 cups |
| 70 | 5 cups | 6 cups | 7 cups |
| 80 | 5 1/2 cups | 6 1/2 cups | 7 1/2 cups |
| 90 | 6 cups | 7 cups | 8 cups |
| 100 | 6 1/2 cups | 7 1/2 cups | 8 1/2 cups |

## Recipe 3: Egg and Veggie Fiesta Bowl

**Ingredients (for 1 cup):**

- 1 large egg (50g)
- 2 tbsp brown rice, cooked (30g)
- 3/4 cup spinach, chopped (75g)
- 1/2 cup carrots, chopped (50g)
- 1/4 cup apples, chopped (25g)
- 1/50 tsp olive oil (0.1g)

- 1 cup water

**Preparation Time:**

- **Prep Time**: 10 minutes
- **Cook Time**: 4 hours
- **Total Time**: 4 hours 10 minutes
- **Difficulty Level**: Easy

**Instructions:**

1. **Prepare the Ingredients**:
    - Cook the brown rice according to package instructions.
    - Chop the spinach, carrots, and apples.
    - Beat the egg lightly.
2. **Combine in the Slow Cooker**:
    - Place the spinach, carrots, apples, and cooked brown rice in the slow cooker.
    - Pour the beaten egg over the vegetable-rice mixture.
    - Add olive oil and water.
3. **Cook**:
    - Set the slow cooker to low and cook for 4 hours or until the vegetables are tender and the egg is fully cooked and mixed with the vegetables and rice.
4. **Cool and Serve**:
    - Allow the mixture to cool to a safe temperature before serving.
    - Portion according to your dog's size and daily caloric needs.

## Nutritional Information (per serving):

| Nutrient | Quantity (per cup) | Daily Value (%) |
|---|---|---|
| Calories | 160 kcal | - |
| Protein | 0.28 oz (7.9 g) | 27.8% |
| Fat | 0.02 oz (0.7 g) | 17.9% |
| Carbohydrates | 0.82 oz (23.8 g) | 53.3% |
| Fiber | 0.06 oz (2.2 g) | 2.5% |

## Suggested Portions (Daily):

| Dog Size (lbs) | Low Activity | Moderate Activity | High Activity |
|---|---|---|---|
| 5 | 1 cup | 1 1/4 cups | 1 1/2 cups |
| 10 | 1 1/2 cups | 2 cups | 2 1/2 cups |
| 20 | 2 1/2 cups | 3 cups | 3 1/2 cups |
| 30 | 3 cups | 4 cups | 4 1/2 cups |
| 40 | 3 1/2 cups | 4 1/2 cups | 5 cups |
| 50 | 4 cups | 5 cups | 6 cups |
| 60 | 4 1/2 cups | 5 1/2 cups | 6 1/2 cups |
| 70 | 5 cups | 6 cups | 7 cups |
| 80 | 5 1/2 cups | 6 1/2 cups | 7 1/2 cups |
| 90 | 6 cups | 7 cups | 8 cups |
| 100 | 6 1/2 cups | 7 1/2 cups | 8 1/2 cups |

## Recipe 4: Wholesome Egg & Veggie Medley

**Ingredients (for 1 cup):**

- 1 large egg (50g)
- 1 tbsp oats, cooked (15g)
- 1/2 cup broccoli, chopped (50g)
- 1/4 cup sweet potatoes, diced (30g)
- 1/4 cup pears, chopped (20g)
- 1/50 tsp olive oil (0.1g)
- 1 cup water

**Preparation Time:**

- **Prep Time**: 10 minutes
- **Cook Time**: 4 hours
- **Total Time**: 4 hours 10 minutes
- **Difficulty Level**: Easy

**Instructions:**

1. **Prepare the Ingredients**:
   - Cook the oats according to package instructions.
   - Chop the broccoli, sweet potatoes, and pears.
   - Beat the egg lightly.
2. **Combine in the Slow Cooker**:
   - Place the broccoli, sweet potatoes, pears, and cooked oats in the slow cooker.
   - Pour the beaten egg over the vegetable-oat mixture.
   - Add olive oil and water.
3. **Cook**:
   - Set the slow cooker to low and cook for 4 hours or until the vegetables are tender and the egg is fully cooked and mixed with the vegetables and oats.
4. **Cool and Serve**:
   - Allow the mixture to cool to a safe temperature before serving.
   - Portion according to your dog's size and daily caloric needs.

## Nutritional Information (per serving):

| Nutrient | Quantity (per cup) | Daily Value (%) |
| --- | --- | --- |
| Calories | 160 kcal | - |
| Protein | 0.24 oz (6.8 g) | 24.0% |
| Fat | 0.01 oz (0.5 g) | 15.0% |
| Carbohydrates | 0.76 oz (21.6 g) | 50.0% |
| Fiber | 0.06 oz (2.6 g) | 2.5% |

## Suggested Portions (Daily):

| Dog Size (lbs) | Low Activity | Moderate Activity | High Activity |
|---|---|---|---|
| 5 | 1 cup | 1 1/4 cups | 1 1/2 cups |
| 10 | 1 1/2 cups | 2 cups | 2 1/2 cups |
| 20 | 2 1/2 cups | 3 cups | 3 1/2 cups |
| 30 | 3 cups | 4 cups | 4 1/2 cups |
| 40 | 3 1/2 cups | 4 1/2 cups | 5 cups |
| 50 | 4 cups | 5 cups | 6 cups |
| 60 | 4 1/2 cups | 5 1/2 cups | 6 1/2 cups |
| 70 | 5 cups | 6 cups | 7 cups |
| 80 | 5 1/2 cups | 6 1/2 cups | 7 1/2 cups |
| 90 | 6 cups | 7 cups | 8 cups |
| 100 | 6 1/2 cups | 7 1/2 cups | 8 1/2 cups |

## Recipe 5: Rainbow Egg & Quinoa Delight

**Ingredients (for 1 cup):**

- 1 large egg (50g)
- 3 tbsp quinoa, cooked (45g)
- 2/3 cup kale, chopped (60g)
- 1/3 cup pumpkin, cooked (50g)
- 1/4 cup strawberries, chopped (35g)
- 1/50 tsp olive oil (0.1g)
- 1 cup water

**Preparation Time:**

- **Prep Time**: 10 minutes
- **Cook Time**: 4 hours
- **Total Time**: 4 hours 10 minutes
- **Difficulty Level**: Easy

**Instructions:**

1. **Prepare the Ingredients**:
    - Cook the quinoa according to package instructions.
    - Chop the kale, pumpkin, and strawberries.
    - Beat the egg lightly.
2. **Combine in the Slow Cooker**:
    - Place the kale, pumpkin, strawberries, and cooked quinoa in the slow cooker.
    - Pour the beaten egg over the vegetable-quinoa mixture.
    - Add olive oil and water.
3. **Cook**:
    - Set the slow cooker to low and cook for 4 hours or until the vegetables are tender and the egg is fully cooked and mixed with the vegetables and quinoa.

4. **Cool and Serve**:
    - Allow the mixture to cool to a safe temperature before serving.
    - Portion according to your dog's size and daily caloric needs.

## Nutritional Information (per serving):

| Nutrient | Quantity (per cup) | Daily Value (%) |
|---|---|---|
| Calories | 160 kcal | - |
| Protein | 0.28 oz (8.1 g) | 26.2% |
| Fat | 0.02 oz (0.6 g) | 15.0% |
| Carbohydrates | 0.80 oz (22.8 g) | 51.8% |
| Fiber | 0.06 oz (2.5 g) | 2.5% |

## Suggested Portions (Daily):

| Dog Size (lbs) | Low Activity | Moderate Activity | High Activity |
|---|---|---|---|
| 5 | 1 cup | 1 1/4 cups | 1 1/2 cups |
| 10 | 1 1/2 cups | 2 cups | 2 1/2 cups |
| 20 | 2 1/2 cups | 3 cups | 3 1/2 cups |
| 30 | 3 cups | 4 cups | 4 1/2 cups |
| 40 | 3 1/2 cups | 4 1/2 cups | 5 cups |
| 50 | 4 cups | 5 cups | 6 cups |
| 60 | 4 1/2 cups | 5 1/2 cups | 6 1/2 cups |
| 70 | 5 cups | 6 cups | 7 cups |
| 80 | 5 1/2 cups | 6 1/2 cups | 7 1/2 cups |
| 90 | 6 cups | 7 cups | 8 cups |
| 100 | 6 1/2 cups | 7 1/2 cups | 8 1/2 cups |

# Liver Recipes

### Recipe 1: Liver & Veggie Delight

**Ingredients (for 1 cup):**

- 1.05 oz chicken liver (30g)
- 2 tbsp brown rice, cooked (30g)
- 1 cup spinach, chopped (100g)
- 3/4 cup carrots, chopped (90g)
- 1/3 cup blueberries, chopped (50g)
- 1/50 tsp olive oil (0.1g)
- 1 cup water

**Preparation Time:**

- **Prep Time**: 10 minutes
- **Cook Time**: 4 hours
- **Total Time**: 4 hours 10 minutes
- **Difficulty Level**: Easy

**Instructions:**

1. **Prepare the Ingredients**:
   - Cook the brown rice according to package instructions.
   - Chop the spinach, carrots, and blueberries.
   - Slice the chicken liver into small pieces.
2. **Combine in the Slow Cooker**:
   - Place the chicken liver, spinach, carrots, blueberries, and cooked brown rice in the slow cooker.
   - Add olive oil and water.
3. **Cook**:
   - Set the slow cooker to low and cook for 4 hours or until the vegetables are tender and the liver is fully cooked.
4. **Cool and Serve**:
   - Allow the mixture to cool to a safe temperature before serving.
   - Portion according to your dog's size and daily caloric needs.

### Nutritional Information (per serving):

| Nutrient | Quantity (per cup) | Daily Value (%) |
|---|---|---|
| Calories | 172 kcal | - |
| Protein | 0.22 oz (6.4 g) | 30.15% |
| Fat | 0.01 oz (0.4 g) | 6.19% |
| Carbohydrates | 0.89 oz (24.5 g) | 63.66% |
| Fiber | 0.07 oz (2.0 g) | 2.0% |

## Suggested Portions (Daily):

| Dog Size (lbs) | Low Activity | Moderate Activity | High Activity |
|---|---|---|---|
| 5 | 1 cup | 1 1/4 cups | 1 1/2 cups |
| 10 | 1 1/2 cups | 2 cups | 2 1/2 cups |
| 20 | 2 1/2 cups | 3 cups | 3 1/2 cups |
| 30 | 3 cups | 4 cups | 4 1/2 cups |
| 40 | 3 1/2 cups | 4 1/2 cups | 5 cups |
| 50 | 4 cups | 5 cups | 6 cups |
| 60 | 4 1/2 cups | 5 1/2 cups | 6 1/2 cups |
| 70 | 5 cups | 6 cups | 7 cups |
| 80 | 5 1/2 cups | 6 1/2 cups | 7 1/2 cups |
| 90 | 6 cups | 7 cups | 8 cups |
| 100 | 6 1/2 cups | 7 1/2 cups | 8 1/2 cups |

## Recipe 2: Liver & Veggie Mix

**Ingredients (for 1 cup):**

- 0.88 oz chicken liver (25g)
- 2 tbsp brown rice, cooked (30g)
- 1/2 cup broccoli, chopped (60g)
- 1/2 cup pumpkin, cooked (60g)
- 1/2 cup apples, chopped (55g)
- 1/10 tsp olive oil (2g)
- 1 cup water

**Preparation Time:**

- **Prep Time**: 10 minutes
- **Cook Time**: 4 hours
- **Total Time**: 4 hours 10 minutes
- **Difficulty Level**: Easy

**Instructions:**

1. **Prepare the Ingredients**:
    - Cook the brown rice according to package instructions.
    - Chop the broccoli, pumpkin, and apples.
    - Slice the chicken liver into small pieces.
2. **Combine in the Slow Cooker**:
    - Place the chicken liver, broccoli, pumpkin, apples, and cooked brown rice in the slow cooker.
    - Add olive oil and water.
3. **Cook**:
    - Set the slow cooker to low and cook for 4 hours or until the vegetables are tender and the liver is fully cooked.
4. **Cool and Serve**:
    - Allow the mixture to cool to a safe temperature before serving.

- Portion according to your dog's size and daily caloric needs.

## Nutritional Information (per serving):

| Nutrient | Quantity (per cup) | Daily Value (%) |
|---|---|---|
| Calories | 164 kcal | - |
| Protein | 0.88 oz (6.1 g) | 25.6% |
| Fat | 0.02 oz (0.7 g) | 10.4% |
| Carbohydrates | 0.88 oz (24.8 g) | 63.9% |
| Fiber | 0.02 oz (1.5 g) | 1.5% |

## Suggested Portions (Daily):

| Dog Size (lbs) | Low Activity | Moderate Activity | High Activity |
|---|---|---|---|
| 5 | 1 cup | 1 1/4 cups | 1 1/2 cups |
| 10 | 1 1/2 cups | 2 cups | 2 1/2 cups |
| 20 | 2 1/2 cups | 3 cups | 3 1/2 cups |
| 30 | 3 cups | 4 cups | 4 1/2 cups |
| 40 | 3 1/2 cups | 4 1/2 cups | 5 cups |
| 50 | 4 cups | 5 cups | 6 cups |
| 60 | 4 1/2 cups | 5 1/2 cups | 6 1/2 cups |
| 70 | 5 cups | 6 cups | 7 cups |
| 80 | 5 1/2 cups | 6 1/2 cups | 7 1/2 cups |
| 90 | 6 cups | 7 cups | 8 cups |
| 100 | 6 1/2 cups | 7 1/2 cups | 8 1/2 cups |

## Recipe 3: Liver & Veggie Power Bowl

**Ingredients (for 1 cup):**

- 0.88 oz chicken liver (25g)
- 2 tbsp brown rice, cooked (30g)
- 1/2 cup spinach, chopped (60g)
- 1/2 cup sweet potatoes, diced (60g)
- 1/2 cup green beans, chopped (55g)
- 1/2 tsp olive oil (2g)
- 1 cup water

**Preparation Time:**

- **Prep Time**: 10 minutes
- **Cook Time**: 4 hours
- **Total Time**: 4 hours 10 minutes
- **Difficulty Level**: Easy

**Instructions:**

1. **Prepare the Ingredients:**
   - Cook the brown rice according to package instructions.
   - Chop the spinach, sweet potatoes, and green beans.
   - Slice the chicken liver into small pieces.
2. **Combine in the Slow Cooker:**
   - Place the chicken liver, spinach, sweet potatoes, green beans, and cooked brown rice in the slow cooker.
   - Add olive oil and water.
3. **Cook:**
   - Set the slow cooker to low and cook for 4 hours or until the vegetables are tender and the liver is fully cooked.
4. **Cool and Serve:**
   - Allow the mixture to cool to a safe temperature before serving.
   - Portion according to your dog's size and daily caloric needs.

## Nutritional Information (per serving):

| Nutrient | Quantity (per cup) | Daily Value (%) |
|---|---|---|
| Calories | 160 kcal | - |
| Protein | 0.88 oz (7.2 g) | 18.0% |
| Fat | 0.02 oz (4.0 g) | 15.0% |
| Carbohydrates | 0.88 oz (16.0 g) | 60.0% |
| Fiber | 0.02 oz (2.5 g) | 4.5% |

## Suggested Portions (Daily):

| Dog Size (lbs) | Low Activity | Moderate Activity | High Activity |
|---|---|---|---|
| 5 | 1 cup | 1 1/4 cups | 1 1/2 cups |
| 10 | 1 1/2 cups | 2 cups | 2 1/2 cups |
| 20 | 2 1/2 cups | 3 cups | 3 1/2 cups |
| 30 | 3 cups | 4 cups | 4 1/2 cups |
| 40 | 3 1/2 cups | 4 1/2 cups | 5 cups |
| 50 | 4 cups | 5 cups | 6 cups |
| 60 | 4 1/2 cups | 5 1/2 cups | 6 1/2 cups |
| 70 | 5 cups | 6 cups | 7 cups |
| 80 | 5 1/2 cups | 6 1/2 cups | 7 1/2 cups |
| 90 | 6 cups | 7 cups | 8 cups |
| 100 | 6 1/2 cups | 7 1/2 cups | 8 1/2 cups |

## Recipe 4: Lamb Liver & Veggie Medley

**Ingredients (for 1 cup):**

- 0.88 oz lamb liver (25g)
- 2 tbsp quinoa, cooked (30g)
- 1/2 cup broccoli, chopped (60g)

- 1/2 cup carrots, chopped (60g)
- 1/2 cup blueberries, chopped (55g)
- 1 tsp olive oil (4g)
- 1 cup water

**Preparation Time:**

- **Prep Time**: 10 minutes
- **Cook Time**: 4 hours
- **Total Time**: 4 hours 10 minutes
- **Difficulty Level**: Easy

**Instructions:**

1. **Prepare the Ingredients**:
    - Cook the quinoa according to package instructions.
    - Chop the broccoli, carrots, and blueberries.
    - Slice the lamb liver into small pieces.
2. **Combine in the Slow Cooker**:
    - Place the lamb liver, quinoa, broccoli, carrots, and blueberries in the slow cooker.
    - Add olive oil and water.
3. **Cook**:
    - Set the slow cooker to low and cook for 4 hours or until the vegetables are tender and the liver is fully cooked.
4. **Cool and Serve**:
    - Allow the mixture to cool to a safe temperature before serving.
    - Portion according to your dog's size and daily caloric needs.

## Nutritional Information (per serving):

| Nutrient | Quantity (per cup) | Daily Value (%) |
|---|---|---|
| Calories | 160 kcal | - |
| Protein | 0.88 oz (7.0 g) | 25.0% |
| Fat | 0.02 oz (6.4 g) | 15.0% |
| Carbohydrates | 0.88 oz (24.0 g) | 60.0% |
| Fiber | 0.02 oz (2.5 g) | 2.5% |

## Suggested Portions (Daily):

| Dog Size (lbs) | Low Activity | Moderate Activity | High Activity |
|---|---|---|---|
| 5 | 1 cup | 1 1/4 cups | 1 1/2 cups |
| 10 | 1 1/2 cups | 2 cups | 2 1/2 cups |
| 20 | 2 1/2 cups | 3 cups | 3 1/2 cups |
| 30 | 3 cups | 4 cups | 4 1/2 cups |
| 40 | 3 1/2 cups | 4 1/2 cups | 5 cups |
| 50 | 4 cups | 5 cups | 6 cups |
| 60 | 4 1/2 cups | 5 1/2 cups | 6 1/2 cups |
| 70 | 5 cups | 6 cups | 7 cups |
| 80 | 5 1/2 cups | 6 1/2 cups | 7 1/2 cups |

| | | | |
|---|---|---|---|
| 90 | 6 cups | 7 cups | 8 cups |
| 100 | 6 1/2 cups | 7 1/2 cups | 8 1/2 cups |

## Recipe 5: Lamb Liver & Veggie Delight

**Ingredients (for 1 cup):**

- 0.88 oz lamb liver (25g)
- 1.5 tbsp oats, cooked (22.5g)
- 1/2 cup zucchini, chopped (60g)
- 1/2 cup peas, cooked (50g)
- 1/2 cup apples, chopped (50g)
- 1/2 tsp olive oil (2g)
- 1 cup water

**Preparation Time:**

- **Prep Time**: 10 minutes
- **Cook Time**: 4 hours
- **Total Time**: 4 hours 10 minutes
- **Difficulty Level**: Easy

**Instructions:**

1. **Prepare the Ingredients**:
   - Cook the oats according to package instructions.
   - Chop the zucchini, peas, and apples.
   - Slice the lamb liver into small pieces.
2. **Combine in the Slow Cooker**:
   - Place the lamb liver, oats, zucchini, peas, and apples in the slow cooker.
   - Add olive oil and water.
3. **Cook**:
   - Set the slow cooker to low and cook for 4 hours or until the vegetables are tender and the liver is fully cooked.
4. **Cool and Serve**:
   - Allow the mixture to cool to a safe temperature before serving.
   - Portion according to your dog's size and daily caloric needs.

## Nutritional Information (per serving):

| Nutrient | Quantity (per cup) | Daily Value (%) |
|---|---|---|
| Calories | 160 kcal | - |
| Protein | 0.88 oz (7.2 g) | 27.0% |
| Fat | 0.02 oz (4.8 g) | 15.0% |
| Carbohydrates | 0.88 oz (15.2 g) | 58.0% |
| Fiber | 0.02 oz (2.5 g) | 2.5% |

## Suggested Portions (Daily):

| Dog Size (lbs) | Low Activity | Moderate Activity | High Activity |
|---|---|---|---|
| 5 | 1 cup | 1 1/4 cups | 1 1/2 cups |
| 10 | 1 1/2 cups | 2 cups | 2 1/2 cups |
| 20 | 2 1/2 cups | 3 cups | 3 1/2 cups |
| 30 | 3 cups | 4 cups | 4 1/2 cups |
| 40 | 3 1/2 cups | 4 1/2 cups | 5 cups |
| 50 | 4 cups | 5 cups | 6 cups |
| 60 | 4 1/2 cups | 5 1/2 cups | 6 1/2 cups |
| 70 | 5 cups | 6 cups | 7 cups |
| 80 | 5 1/2 cups | 6 1/2 cups | 7 1/2 cups |
| 90 | 6 cups | 7 cups | 8 cups |
| 100 | 6 1/2 cups | 7 1/2 cups | 8 1/2 cups |

# Heart Recipes

## Recipe 1: Beef Heart & Veggie Feast

**Ingredients (for 1 cup):**

- 0.88 oz beef heart (25g)
- 2 tbsp brown rice, cooked (20g)
- 1/2 cup carrots, chopped (60g)
- 1/2 cup spinach, chopped (60g)
- 1/2 cup blueberries, chopped (55g)
- 1 tsp olive oil (4g)
- 1 cup water

**Preparation Time:**

- **Prep Time**: 10 minutes
- **Cook Time**: 4 hours
- **Total Time**: 4 hours 10 minutes
- **Difficulty Level**: Easy

**Instructions:**

1. **Prepare the Ingredients**:
   - Cook the brown rice according to package instructions.
   - Chop the carrots, spinach, and blueberries.
   - Slice the beef heart into small pieces.
2. **Combine in the Slow Cooker**:
   - Place the beef heart, brown rice, carrots, spinach, and blueberries in the slow cooker.
   - Add olive oil and water.
3. **Cook**:
   - Set the slow cooker to low and cook for 4 hours or until the vegetables are tender and the heart is fully cooked.
4. **Cool and Serve**:
   - Allow the mixture to cool to a safe temperature before serving.
   - Portion according to your dog's size and daily caloric needs.

### Nutritional Information (per serving):

| Nutrient | Quantity (per cup) | Daily Value (%) |
|---|---|---|
| Calories | 160 kcal | - |
| Protein | 0.88 oz (7.5 g) | 24.0% |
| Fat | 0.02 oz (6.0 g) | 13.5% |
| Carbohydrates | 0.88 oz (16.0 g) | 56.0% |
| Fiber | 0.02 oz (2.5 g) | 2.5% |

## Suggested Portions (Daily):

| Dog Size (lbs) | Low Activity | Moderate Activity | High Activity |
|---|---|---|---|
| 5 | 1 cup | 1 1/4 cups | 1 1/2 cups |
| 10 | 1 1/2 cups | 2 cups | 2 1/2 cups |
| 20 | 2 1/2 cups | 3 cups | 3 1/2 cups |
| 30 | 3 cups | 4 cups | 4 1/2 cups |
| 40 | 3 1/2 cups | 4 1/2 cups | 5 cups |
| 50 | 4 cups | 5 cups | 6 cups |
| 60 | 4 1/2 cups | 5 1/2 cups | 6 1/2 cups |
| 70 | 5 cups | 6 cups | 7 cups |
| 80 | 5 1/2 cups | 6 1/2 cups | 7 1/2 cups |
| 90 | 6 cups | 7 cups | 8 cups |
| 100 | 6 1/2 cups | 7 1/2 cups | 8 1/2 cups |

## Recipe 2: Chicken Heart & Veggie Delight

**Ingredients (for 1 cup):**

- 0.88 oz chicken heart (25g)
- 2 tbsp quinoa, cooked (30g)
- 1/2 cup carrots, chopped (60g)
- 1/2 cup broccoli, chopped (60g)
- 1/4 cup apples, chopped (30g)
- 1 tsp olive oil (4g)
- 1 cup water

**Preparation Time:**

- **Prep Time**: 10 minutes
- **Cook Time**: 4 hours
- **Total Time**: 4 hours 10 minutes
- **Difficulty Level**: Easy

**Instructions:**

1. **Prepare the Ingredients**:
    - Cook the quinoa according to package instructions.
    - Chop the carrots, broccoli, and apples.
    - Slice the chicken heart into small pieces.
2. **Combine in the Slow Cooker**:
    - Place the chicken heart, quinoa, carrots, broccoli, and apples in the slow cooker.
    - Add olive oil and water.
3. **Cook**:
    - Set the slow cooker to low and cook for 4 hours or until the vegetables are tender and the heart is fully cooked.
4. **Cool and Serve**:
    - Allow the mixture to cool to a safe temperature before serving.

- Portion according to your dog's size and daily caloric needs.

## Nutritional Information (per serving):

| Nutrient | Quantity (per cup) | Daily Value (%) |
|---|---|---|
| Calories | 160 kcal | - |
| Protein | 0.88 oz (7.5 g) | 22.5% |
| Fat | 0.02 oz (6.0 g) | 15.0% |
| Carbohydrates | 0.88 oz (16.0 g) | 60.0% |
| Fiber | 0.02 oz (2.5 g) | 2.5% |

## Suggested Portions (Daily):

| Dog Size (lbs) | Low Activity | Moderate Activity | High Activity |
|---|---|---|---|
| 5 | 1 cup | 1 1/4 cups | 1 1/2 cups |
| 10 | 1 1/2 cups | 2 cups | 2 1/2 cups |
| 20 | 2 1/2 cups | 3 cups | 3 1/2 cups |
| 30 | 3 cups | 4 cups | 4 1/2 cups |
| 40 | 3 1/2 cups | 4 1/2 cups | 5 cups |
| 50 | 4 cups | 5 cups | 6 cups |
| 60 | 4 1/2 cups | 5 1/2 cups | 6 1/2 cups |
| 70 | 5 cups | 6 cups | 7 cups |
| 80 | 5 1/2 cups | 6 1/2 cups | 7 1/2 cups |
| 90 | 6 cups | 7 cups | 8 cups |
| 100 | 6 1/2 cups | 7 1/2 cups | 8 1/2 cups |

## Recipe 3: Turkey Heart & Autumn Veggie Feast

### Ingredients (for 1 cup):

- 0.88 oz turkey heart (25g)
- 2 tbsp brown rice, cooked (30g)
- 1/2 cup butternut squash, diced (60g)
- 1/2 cup green beans, chopped (60g)
- 1/4 cup cranberries, chopped (30g)
- 1 tsp olive oil (4g)
- 1 cup water

### Preparation Time:

- **Prep Time**: 10 minutes
- **Cook Time**: 4 hours
- **Total Time**: 4 hours 10 minutes
- **Difficulty Level**: Easy

**Instructions:**

1. **Prepare the Ingredients:**
    - Cook the brown rice according to package instructions.
    - Chop the butternut squash, green beans, and cranberries.
    - Slice the turkey heart into small pieces.
2. **Combine in the Slow Cooker:**
    - Place the turkey heart, brown rice, butternut squash, green beans, and cranberries in the slow cooker.
    - Add olive oil and water.
3. **Cook:**
    - Set the slow cooker to low and cook for 4 hours or until the vegetables are tender and the heart is fully cooked.
4. **Cool and Serve:**
    - Allow the mixture to cool to a safe temperature before serving.
    - Portion according to your dog's size and daily caloric needs.

### Nutritional Information (per serving):

| Nutrient | Quantity (per cup) | Daily Value (%) |
|---|---|---|
| Calories | 160 kcal | - |
| Protein | 0.88 oz (7.5 g) | 22.5% |
| Fat | 0.02 oz (6.0 g) | 15.0% |
| Carbohydrates | 0.88 oz (16.0 g) | 60.0% |
| Fiber | 0.02 oz (2.5 g) | 2.5% |

### Suggested Portions (Daily):

| Dog Size (lbs) | Low Activity | Moderate Activity | High Activity |
|---|---|---|---|
| 5 | 1 cup | 1 1/4 cups | 1 1/2 cups |
| 10 | 1 1/2 cups | 2 cups | 2 1/2 cups |
| 20 | 2 1/2 cups | 3 cups | 3 1/2 cups |
| 30 | 3 cups | 4 cups | 4 1/2 cups |
| 40 | 3 1/2 cups | 4 1/2 cups | 5 cups |
| 50 | 4 cups | 5 cups | 6 cups |
| 60 | 4 1/2 cups | 5 1/2 cups | 6 1/2 cups |
| 70 | 5 cups | 6 cups | 7 cups |
| 80 | 5 1/2 cups | 6 1/2 cups | 7 1/2 cups |
| 90 | 6 cups | 7 cups | 8 cups |
| 100 | 6 1/2 cups | 7 1/2 cups | 8 1/2 cups |

### Recipe 4: Lamb Heart & Garden Veggie Delight

**Ingredients (for 1 cup):**

- 0.88 oz lamb heart (25g)
- 2 tbsp quinoa, cooked (30g)
- 1/2 cup zucchini, chopped (60g)

- 1/2 cup sweet potatoes, diced (60g)
- 1/4 cup cranberries, chopped (30g)
- 1 tsp olive oil (4g)
- 1 cup water

**Preparation Time:**

- **Prep Time**: 10 minutes
- **Cook Time**: 4 hours
- **Total Time**: 4 hours 10 minutes
- **Difficulty Level**: Easy

**Instructions:**

1. **Prepare the Ingredients**:
   - Cook the quinoa according to package instructions.
   - Chop the zucchini, sweet potatoes, and cranberries.
   - Slice the lamb heart into small pieces.
2. **Combine in the Slow Cooker**:
   - Place the lamb heart, quinoa, zucchini, sweet potatoes, and cranberries in the slow cooker.
   - Add olive oil and water.
3. **Cook**:
   - Set the slow cooker to low and cook for 4 hours or until the vegetables are tender and the heart is fully cooked.
4. **Cool and Serve**:
   - Allow the mixture to cool to a safe temperature before serving.
   - Portion according to your dog's size and daily caloric needs.

## Nutritional Information (per serving):

| Nutrient | Quantity (per cup) | Daily Value (%) |
|---|---|---|
| Calories | 160 kcal | - |
| Protein | 0.88 oz (7.2 g) | 24.0% |
| Fat | 0.02 oz (6.0 g) | 15.0% |
| Carbohydrates | 0.88 oz (16.0 g) | 56.0% |
| Fiber | 0.02 oz (2.5 g) | 2.5% |

## Suggested Portions (Daily):

| Dog Size (lbs) | Low Activity | Moderate Activity | High Activity |
|---|---|---|---|
| 5 | 1 cup | 1 1/4 cups | 1 1/2 cups |
| 10 | 1 1/2 cups | 2 cups | 2 1/2 cups |
| 20 | 2 1/2 cups | 3 cups | 3 1/2 cups |
| 30 | 3 cups | 4 cups | 4 1/2 cups |
| 40 | 3 1/2 cups | 4 1/2 cups | 5 cups |
| 50 | 4 cups | 5 cups | 6 cups |
| 60 | 4 1/2 cups | 5 1/2 cups | 6 1/2 cups |
| 70 | 5 cups | 6 cups | 7 cups |
| 80 | 5 1/2 cups | 6 1/2 cups | 7 1/2 cups |
| 90 | 6 cups | 7 cups | 8 cups |
| 100 | 6 1/2 cups | 7 1/2 cups | 8 1/2 cups |

## Recipe 5: Chicken Heart & Veggie Harvest Feast

**Ingredients (for 1 cup):**

- 0.88 oz chicken heart (25g)
- 2 tbsp brown rice, cooked (30g)
- 1/2 cup kale, chopped (60g)
- 1/2 cup pumpkin, cooked and mashed (60g)
- 1/4 cup blueberries, chopped (30g)
- 1 tsp olive oil (4g)
- 1 cup water

**Preparation Time:**

- **Prep Time**: 10 minutes
- **Cook Time**: 4 hours
- **Total Time**: 4 hours 10 minutes
- **Difficulty Level**: Easy

**Instructions:**

1. **Prepare the Ingredients**:
    - Cook the brown rice according to package instructions.
    - Chop the kale, pumpkin, and blueberries.
    - Slice the chicken heart into small pieces.
2. **Combine in the Slow Cooker**:
    - Place the chicken heart, brown rice, kale, pumpkin, and blueberries in the slow cooker.
    - Add olive oil and water.
3. **Cook**:
    - Set the slow cooker to low and cook for 4 hours or until the vegetables are tender and the heart is fully cooked.
4. **Cool and Serve**:
    - Allow the mixture to cool to a safe temperature before serving.

- Portion according to your dog's size and daily caloric needs.

## Nutritional Information (per serving):

| Nutrient | Quantity (per cup) | Daily Value (%) |
|---|---|---|
| Calories | 160 kcal | - |
| Protein | 0.88 oz (7.5 g) | 24.0% |
| Fat | 0.02 oz (6.0 g) | 15.0% |
| Carbohydrates | 0.88 oz (16.0 g) | 56.0% |
| Fiber | 0.02 oz (2.5 g) | 2.5% |

## Suggested Portions (Daily):

| Dog Size (lbs) | Low Activity | Moderate Activity | High Activity |
|---|---|---|---|
| 5 | 1 cup | 1 1/4 cups | 1 1/2 cups |
| 10 | 1 1/2 cups | 2 cups | 2 1/2 cups |
| 20 | 2 1/2 cups | 3 cups | 3 1/2 cups |
| 30 | 3 cups | 4 cups | 4 1/2 cups |
| 40 | 3 1/2 cups | 4 1/2 cups | 5 cups |
| 50 | 4 cups | 5 cups | 6 cups |
| 60 | 4 1/2 cups | 5 1/2 cups | 6 1/2 cups |
| 70 | 5 cups | 6 cups | 7 cups |
| 80 | 5 1/2 cups | 6 1/2 cups | 7 1/2 cups |
| 90 | 6 cups | 7 cups | 8 cups |
| 100 | 6 1/2 cups | 7 1/2 cups | 8 1/2 cups |

# Salmon Recipes

### Recipe 1: Salmon & Veggie Delight

**Ingredients (for 1 cup):**

- 0.70 oz salmon (20g)
- 2 tbsp quinoa, cooked (20g)
- 1/2 cup sweet potatoes, diced (60g)
- 1/2 cup spinach, chopped (60g)
- 1/4 cup blueberries, chopped (40g)
- 1/2 tsp olive oil (2g)
- 1 cup water

**Preparation Time:**

- **Prep Time**: 10 minutes
- **Cook Time**: 4 hours
- **Total Time**: 4 hours 10 minutes
- **Difficulty Level**: Easy

**Instructions:**

1. **Prepare the Ingredients**:
    - Cook the quinoa according to package instructions.
    - Chop the sweet potatoes, spinach, and blueberries.
    - Cut the salmon into small pieces.
2. **Combine in the Slow Cooker**:
    - Place the salmon, quinoa, sweet potatoes, spinach, and blueberries in the slow cooker.
    - Add olive oil and water.
3. **Cook**:
    - Set the slow cooker to low and cook for 4 hours or until the vegetables are tender and the salmon is fully cooked.
4. **Cool and Serve**:
    - Allow the mixture to cool to a safe temperature before serving.
    - Portion according to your dog's size and daily caloric needs.

### Nutritional Information (per serving):

| Nutrient | Quantity (per cup) | Daily Value (%) |
|---|---|---|
| Calories | 160 kcal | - |
| Protein | 0.88 oz (7.2 g) | 18% |
| Fat | 0.02 oz (4.8 g) | 12% |
| Carbohydrates | 0.88 oz (24.0 g) | 60% |
| Fiber | 0.02 oz (2.5 g) | 2.5% |

## Suggested Portions (Daily):

| Dog Size (lbs) | Low Activity | Moderate Activity | High Activity |
|---|---|---|---|
| 5 | 1 cup | 1 1/4 cups | 1 1/2 cups |
| 10 | 1 1/2 cups | 2 cups | 2 1/2 cups |
| 20 | 2 1/2 cups | 3 cups | 3 1/2 cups |
| 30 | 3 cups | 4 cups | 4 1/2 cups |
| 40 | 3 1/2 cups | 4 1/2 cups | 5 cups |
| 50 | 4 cups | 5 cups | 6 cups |
| 60 | 4 1/2 cups | 5 1/2 cups | 6 1/2 cups |
| 70 | 5 cups | 6 cups | 7 cups |
| 80 | 5 1/2 cups | 6 1/2 cups | 7 1/2 cups |
| 90 | 6 cups | 7 cups | 8 cups |
| 100 | 6 1/2 cups | 7 1/2 cups | 8 1/2 cups |

## Recipe 2: Salmon & Garden Veggie Delight

**Ingredients (for 1 cup):**

- 0.53 oz salmon (15g)
- 2 tbsp brown rice, cooked (20g)
- 1/2 cup green beans, chopped (60g)
- 1/2 cup carrots, chopped (60g)
- 1/4 cup apples, chopped (40g)
- 1/4 tsp olive oil (1g)
- 1 cup water

**Preparation Time:**

- **Prep Time**: 10 minutes
- **Cook Time**: 4 hours
- **Total Time**: 4 hours 10 minutes
- **Difficulty Level**: Easy

**Instructions:**

1. **Prepare the Ingredients**:
   - Cook the brown rice according to package instructions.
   - Chop the green beans, carrots, and apples.
   - Cut the salmon into small pieces.
2. **Combine in the Slow Cooker**:
   - Place the salmon, brown rice, green beans, carrots, and apples in the slow cooker.
   - Add olive oil and water.
3. **Cook**:
   - Set the slow cooker to low and cook for 4 hours or until the vegetables are tender and the salmon is fully cooked.
4. **Cool and Serve**:
   - Allow the mixture to cool to a safe temperature before serving.
   - Portion according to your dog's size and daily caloric needs.

## Nutritional Information (per serving):

| Nutrient | Quantity (per cup) | Daily Value (%) |
|---|---|---|
| Calories | 160 kcal | - |
| Protein | 0.53 oz (5.4 g) | 19% |
| Fat | 0.01 oz (3.1 g) | 12% |
| Carbohydrates | 0.88 oz (22.0 g) | 56% |
| Fiber | 0.02 oz (2.5 g) | 2.5% |

## Suggested Portions (Daily):

| Dog Size (lbs) | Low Activity | Moderate Activity | High Activity |
|---|---|---|---|
| 5 | 1 cup | 1 1/4 cups | 1 1/2 cups |
| 10 | 1 1/2 cups | 2 cups | 2 1/2 cups |
| 20 | 2 1/2 cups | 3 cups | 3 1/2 cups |
| 30 | 3 cups | 4 cups | 4 1/2 cups |
| 40 | 3 1/2 cups | 4 1/2 cups | 5 cups |
| 50 | 4 cups | 5 cups | 6 cups |
| 60 | 4 1/2 cups | 5 1/2 cups | 6 1/2 cups |
| 70 | 5 cups | 6 cups | 7 cups |
| 80 | 5 1/2 cups | 6 1/2 cups | 7 1/2 cups |
| 90 | 6 cups | 7 cups | 8 cups |
| 100 | 6 1/2 cups | 7 1/2 cups | 8 1/2 cups |

## Recipe 3: Salmon & Veggie Harvest Feast

**Ingredients (for 1 cup):**

- 0.53 oz salmon (15g)
- 2 tbsp oats, cooked (15g)
- 1/2 cup broccoli, chopped (60g)
- 1/2 cup peas (60g)
- 1/4 cup strawberries, chopped (40g)
- 1/4 tsp olive oil (1g)
- 1 cup water

**Preparation Time:**

- **Prep Time**: 10 minutes
- **Cook Time**: 4 hours
- **Total Time**: 4 hours 10 minutes
- **Difficulty Level**: Easy

**Instructions:**

1. **Prepare the Ingredients**:
    - Cook the oats according to package instructions.
    - Chop the broccoli, peas, and strawberries.

o Cut the salmon into small pieces.
2. **Combine in the Slow Cooker**:
   o Place the salmon, oats, broccoli, peas, and strawberries in the slow cooker.
   o Add olive oil and water.
3. **Cook**:
   o Set the slow cooker to low and cook for 4 hours or until the vegetables are tender and the salmon is fully cooked.
4. **Cool and Serve**:
   o Allow the mixture to cool to a safe temperature before serving.
   o Portion according to your dog's size and daily caloric needs.

## Nutritional Information (per serving):

| Nutrient | Quantity (per cup) | Daily Value (%) |
|---|---|---|
| Calories | 160 kcal | - |
| Protein | 0.53 oz (5.4 g) | 20% |
| Fat | 0.01 oz (2.7 g) | 15% |
| Carbohydrates | 0.88 oz (21.3 g) | 53% |
| Fiber | 0.02 oz (2.5 g) | 2.5% |

## Suggested Portions (Daily):

| Dog Size (lbs) | Low Activity | Moderate Activity | High Activity |
|---|---|---|---|
| 5 | 1 cup | 1 1/4 cups | 1 1/2 cups |
| 10 | 1 1/2 cups | 2 cups | 2 1/2 cups |
| 20 | 2 1/2 cups | 3 cups | 3 1/2 cups |
| 30 | 3 cups | 4 cups | 4 1/2 cups |
| 40 | 3 1/2 cups | 4 1/2 cups | 5 cups |
| 50 | 4 cups | 5 cups | 6 cups |
| 60 | 4 1/2 cups | 5 1/2 cups | 6 1/2 cups |
| 70 | 5 cups | 6 cups | 7 cups |
| 80 | 5 1/2 cups | 6 1/2 cups | 7 1/2 cups |
| 90 | 6 cups | 7 cups | 8 cups |
| 100 | 6 1/2 cups | 7 1/2 cups | 8 1/2 cups |

## Recipe 4: Salmon & Sweet Potato Medley

**Ingredients (for 1 cup):**

- 0.53 oz salmon (15g)
- 1/3 cup sweet potatoes, diced (40g)
- 1/3 cup kale, chopped (40g)
- 1/3 cup pumpkin, cooked and mashed (40g)
- 1/4 cup blueberries, chopped (30g)
- 1/4 tsp olive oil (1g)
- 1 cup water

**Preparation Time:**

- **Prep Time**: 10 minutes
- **Cook Time**: 4 hours
- **Total Time**: 4 hours 10 minutes
- **Difficulty Level**: Easy

**Instructions:**

1. **Prepare the Ingredients**:
   - Chop the sweet potatoes, kale, pumpkin, and blueberries.
   - Cut the salmon into small pieces.
2. **Combine in the Slow Cooker**:
   - Place the salmon, sweet potatoes, kale, pumpkin, and blueberries in the slow cooker.
   - Add olive oil and water.
3. **Cook**:
   - Set the slow cooker to low and cook for 4 hours or until the vegetables are tender and the salmon is fully cooked.
4. **Cool and Serve**:
   - Allow the mixture to cool to a safe temperature before serving.
   - Portion according to your dog's size and daily caloric needs.

## Nutritional Information (per serving):

| Nutrient | Quantity (per cup) | Daily Value (%) |
|---|---|---|
| Calories | 160 kcal | - |
| Protein | 0.53 oz (5.4 g) | 20% |
| Fat | 0.01 oz (2.7 g) | 15% |
| Carbohydrates | 0.88 oz (21.3 g) | 53% |
| Fiber | 0.02 oz (2.5 g) | 2.5% |

## Suggested Portions (Daily):

| Dog Size (lbs) | Low Activity | Moderate Activity | High Activity |
|---|---|---|---|
| 5 | 1 cup | 1 1/4 cups | 1 1/2 cups |
| 10 | 1 1/2 cups | 2 cups | 2 1/2 cups |
| 20 | 2 1/2 cups | 3 cups | 3 1/2 cups |
| 30 | 3 cups | 4 cups | 4 1/2 cups |
| 40 | 3 1/2 cups | 4 1/2 cups | 5 cups |
| 50 | 4 cups | 5 cups | 6 cups |
| 60 | 4 1/2 cups | 5 1/2 cups | 6 1/2 cups |
| 70 | 5 cups | 6 cups | 7 cups |
| 80 | 5 1/2 cups | 6 1/2 cups | 7 1/2 cups |
| 90 | 6 cups | 7 cups | 8 cups |
| 100 | 6 1/2 cups | 7 1/2 cups | 8 1/2 cups |

## Recipe 5: Salmon & Spinach Supreme

**Ingredients (for 1 cup):**

- 0.53 oz salmon (15g)
- 2 tbsp brown rice, cooked (20g)
- 1/2 cup spinach, chopped (60g)
- 1/2 cup carrots, chopped (60g)
- 1/4 cup apples, chopped (30g)
- 1/4 tsp olive oil (1g)
- 1 cup water

**Preparation Time:**

- **Prep Time**: 10 minutes
- **Cook Time**: 4 hours
- **Total Time**: 4 hours 10 minutes
- **Difficulty Level**: Easy

**Instructions:**

1. **Prepare the Ingredients**:
   - Cook the brown rice according to package instructions.
   - Chop the spinach, carrots, and apples.
   - Cut the salmon into small pieces.
2. **Combine in the Slow Cooker**:
   - Place the salmon, brown rice, spinach, carrots, and apples in the slow cooker.
   - Add olive oil and water.
3. **Cook**:
   - Set the slow cooker to low and cook for 4 hours or until the vegetables are tender and the salmon is fully cooked.
4. **Cool and Serve**:
   - Allow the mixture to cool to a safe temperature before serving.
   - Portion according to your dog's size and daily caloric needs.

### Nutritional Information (per serving):

| Nutrient | Quantity (per cup) | Daily Value (%) |
|---|---|---|
| Calories | 160 kcal | - |
| Protein | 0.53 oz (5.4 g) | 20% |
| Fat | 0.01 oz (2.7 g) | 15% |
| Carbohydrates | 0.88 oz (21.3 g) | 53% |
| Fiber | 0.02 oz (2.5 g) | 2.5% |

## Suggested Portions (Daily):

| Dog Size (lbs) | Low Activity | Moderate Activity | High Activity |
|---|---|---|---|
| 5 | 1 cup | 1 1/4 cups | 1 1/2 cups |
| 10 | 1 1/2 cups | 2 cups | 2 1/2 cups |
| 20 | 2 1/2 cups | 3 cups | 3 1/2 cups |
| 30 | 3 cups | 4 cups | 4 1/2 cups |
| 40 | 3 1/2 cups | 4 1/2 cups | 5 cups |
| 50 | 4 cups | 5 cups | 6 cups |
| 60 | 4 1/2 cups | 5 1/2 cups | 6 1/2 cups |
| 70 | 5 cups | 6 cups | 7 cups |
| 80 | 5 1/2 cups | 6 1/2 cups | 7 1/2 cups |
| 90 | 6 cups | 7 cups | 8 cups |
| 100 | 6 1/2 cups | 7 1/2 cups | 8 1/2 cups |

# Code Recipes

### Recipe 1: Cod & Veggie Delight

**Ingredients (for 1 cup):**

- 1 oz cod (30g)
- 2 tbsp brown rice, cooked (20g)
- 1/2 cup broccoli, chopped (60g)
- 1/2 cup carrots, chopped (60g)
- 1/3 cup apples, chopped (40g)
- 1/2 tsp olive oil (2.5g)
- 1 cup water

**Preparation Time:**

- **Prep Time**: 10 minutes
- **Cook Time**: 4 hours
- **Total Time**: 4 hours 10 minutes
- **Difficulty Level**: Easy

**Instructions:**

1. **Prepare the Ingredients**:
   - Cook the brown rice according to package instructions.
   - Chop the broccoli, carrots, and apples.
   - Cut the cod into small pieces.
2. **Combine in the Slow Cooker**:
   - Place the cod, brown rice, broccoli, carrots, and apples in the slow cooker.
   - Add olive oil and water.
3. **Cook**:
   - Set the slow cooker to low and cook for 4 hours or until the vegetables are tender and the cod is fully cooked.
4. **Cool and Serve**:
   - Allow the mixture to cool to a safe temperature before serving.
   - Portion according to your dog's size and daily caloric needs.

### Nutritional Information (per serving):

| Nutrient | Quantity (per cup) | Daily Value (%) |
|---|---|---|
| Calories | 160 kcal | - |
| Protein | 0.56 oz (7.2 g) | 20% |
| Fat | 0.02 oz (3.0 g) | 15% |
| Carbohydrates | 0.88 oz (21.3 g) | 53% |
| Fiber | 0.02 oz (2.5 g) | 2.5% |

## Suggested Portions (Daily):

| Dog Size (lbs) | Low Activity | Moderate Activity | High Activity |
| --- | --- | --- | --- |
| 5 | 1 cup | 1 1/4 cups | 1 1/2 cups |
| 10 | 1 1/2 cups | 2 cups | 2 1/2 cups |
| 20 | 2 1/2 cups | 3 cups | 3 1/2 cups |
| 30 | 3 cups | 4 cups | 4 1/2 cups |
| 40 | 3 1/2 cups | 4 1/2 cups | 5 cups |
| 50 | 4 cups | 5 cups | 6 cups |
| 60 | 4 1/2 cups | 5 1/2 cups | 6 1/2 cups |
| 70 | 5 cups | 6 cups | 7 cups |
| 80 | 5 1/2 cups | 6 1/2 cups | 7 1/2 cups |
| 90 | 6 cups | 7 cups | 8 cups |
| 100 | 6 1/2 cups | 7 1/2 cups | 8 1/2 cups |

## Recipe 2: Cod & Quinoa Delight

**Ingredients (for 1 cup):**

- 1 oz cod (30g)
- 2 tbsp quinoa, cooked (20g)
- 1/2 cup zucchini, chopped (60g)
- 1/3 cup sweet potatoes, diced (40g)
- 1/4 cup blueberries, chopped (30g)
- 1/2 tsp olive oil (2.5g)
- 1 cup water

**Preparation Time:**

- **Prep Time**: 10 minutes
- **Cook Time**: 4 hours
- **Total Time**: 4 hours 10 minutes
- **Difficulty Level**: Easy

**Instructions:**

1. **Prepare the Ingredients**:
    - Cook the quinoa according to package instructions.
    - Chop the zucchini, sweet potatoes, and blueberries.
    - Cut the cod into small pieces.
2. **Combine in the Slow Cooker**:
    - Place the cod, quinoa, zucchini, sweet potatoes, and blueberries in the slow cooker.
    - Add olive oil and water.
3. **Cook**:
    - Set the slow cooker to low and cook for 4 hours or until the vegetables are tender and the cod is fully cooked.

4. **Cool and Serve**:
    - Allow the mixture to cool to a safe temperature before serving.
    - Portion according to your dog's size and daily caloric needs.

## Nutritional Information (per serving):

| Nutrient | Quantity (per cup) | Daily Value (%) |
|---|---|---|
| Calories | 160 kcal | - |
| Protein | 0.56 oz (7.2 g) | 20% |
| Fat | 0.02 oz (3.0 g) | 15% |
| Carbohydrates | 0.88 oz (21.3 g) | 53% |
| Fiber | 0.02 oz (2.5 g) | 2.5% |

## Suggested Portions (Daily):

| Dog Size (lbs) | Low Activity | Moderate Activity | High Activity |
|---|---|---|---|
| 5 | 1 cup | 1 1/4 cups | 1 1/2 cups |
| 10 | 1 1/2 cups | 2 cups | 2 1/2 cups |
| 20 | 2 1/2 cups | 3 cups | 3 1/2 cups |
| 30 | 3 cups | 4 cups | 4 1/2 cups |
| 40 | 3 1/2 cups | 4 1/2 cups | 5 cups |
| 50 | 4 cups | 5 cups | 6 cups |
| 60 | 4 1/2 cups | 5 1/2 cups | 6 1/2 cups |
| 70 | 5 cups | 6 cups | 7 cups |
| 80 | 5 1/2 cups | 6 1/2 cups | 7 1/2 cups |
| 90 | 6 cups | 7 cups | 8 cups |
| 100 | 6 1/2 cups | 7 1/2 cups | 8 1/2 cups |

## Recipe 3: Cod & Spinach Delight

**Ingredients (for 1 cup):**

- 0.88 oz cod (25g)
- 1 tbsp oats, cooked (10g)
- 1/2 cup spinach, chopped (60g)
- 1/2 cup pumpkin, cooked and mashed (60g)
- 1/3 cup apples, chopped (40g)
- 1/2 tsp olive oil (2.5g)
- 1 cup water

**Preparation Time:**

- **Prep Time**: 10 minutes
- **Cook Time**: 4 hours
- **Total Time**: 4 hours 10 minutes
- **Difficulty Level**: Easy

**Instructions:**

1. **Prepare the Ingredients:**
   - Cook the oats according to package instructions.
   - Chop the spinach, pumpkin, and apples.
   - Cut the cod into small pieces.
2. **Combine in the Slow Cooker:**
   - Place the cod, oats, spinach, pumpkin, and apples in the slow cooker.
   - Add olive oil and water.
3. **Cook:**
   - Set the slow cooker to low and cook for 4 hours or until the vegetables are tender and the cod is fully cooked.
4. **Cool and Serve:**
   - Allow the mixture to cool to a safe temperature before serving.
   - Portion according to your dog's size and daily caloric needs.

## Nutritional Information (per serving):

| Nutrient | Quantity (per cup) | Daily Value (%) |
|---|---|---|
| Calories | 160 kcal | - |
| Protein | 0.44 oz (5.6 g) | 20% |
| Fat | 0.01 oz (3.0 g) | 15% |
| Carbohydrates | 0.88 oz (21.3 g) | 53% |
| Fiber | 0.02 oz (2.5 g) | 2.5% |

## Suggested Portions (Daily):

| Dog Size (lbs) | Low Activity | Moderate Activity | High Activity |
|---|---|---|---|
| 5 | 1 cup | 1 1/4 cups | 1 1/2 cups |
| 10 | 1 1/2 cups | 2 cups | 2 1/2 cups |
| 20 | 2 1/2 cups | 3 cups | 3 1/2 cups |
| 30 | 3 cups | 4 cups | 4 1/2 cups |
| 40 | 3 1/2 cups | 4 1/2 cups | 5 cups |
| 50 | 4 cups | 5 cups | 6 cups |
| 60 | 4 1/2 cups | 5 1/2 cups | 6 1/2 cups |
| 70 | 5 cups | 6 cups | 7 cups |
| 80 | 5 1/2 cups | 6 1/2 cups | 7 1/2 cups |
| 90 | 6 cups | 7 cups | 8 cups |
| 100 | 6 1/2 cups | 7 1/2 cups | 8 1/2 cups |

## Recipe 4: Cod & Kale Delight

**Ingredients (for 1 cup):**

- 1 oz cod (30g)
- 2 tbsp brown rice, cooked (20g)

- 1/2 cup kale, chopped (60g)
- 1/2 cup carrots, chopped (60g)
- 1/3 cup blueberries, chopped (40g)
- 1/2 tsp olive oil (2.5g)
- 1 cup water

**Preparation Time:**

- **Prep Time**: 10 minutes
- **Cook Time**: 4 hours
- **Total Time**: 4 hours 10 minutes
- **Difficulty Level**: Easy

**Instructions:**

1. **Prepare the Ingredients**:
   - Cook the brown rice according to package instructions.
   - Chop the kale, carrots, and blueberries.
   - Cut the cod into small pieces.
2. **Combine in the Slow Cooker**:
   - Place the cod, brown rice, kale, carrots, and blueberries in the slow cooker.
   - Add olive oil and water.
3. **Cook**:
   - Set the slow cooker to low and cook for 4 hours or until the vegetables are tender and the cod is fully cooked.
4. **Cool and Serve**:
   - Allow the mixture to cool to a safe temperature before serving.
   - Portion according to your dog's size and daily caloric needs.

## Nutritional Information (per serving):

| Nutrient | Quantity (per cup) | Daily Value (%) |
|---|---|---|
| Calories | 160 kcal | - |
| Protein | 0.51 oz (6.5 g) | 20% |
| Fat | 0.01 oz (3.2 g) | 15% |
| Carbohydrates | 0.88 oz (21.3 g) | 53% |
| Fiber | 0.02 oz (2.5 g) | 2.5% |

## Suggested Portions (Daily):

| Dog Size (lbs) | Low Activity | Moderate Activity | High Activity |
|---|---|---|---|
| 5 | 1 cup | 1 1/4 cups | 1 1/2 cups |
| 10 | 1 1/2 cups | 2 cups | 2 1/2 cups |
| 20 | 2 1/2 cups | 3 cups | 3 1/2 cups |
| 30 | 3 cups | 4 cups | 4 1/2 cups |
| 40 | 3 1/2 cups | 4 1/2 cups | 5 cups |
| 50 | 4 cups | 5 cups | 6 cups |
| 60 | 4 1/2 cups | 5 1/2 cups | 6 1/2 cups |
| 70 | 5 cups | 6 cups | 7 cups |

| 80 | 5 1/2 cups | 6 1/2 cups | 7 1/2 cups |
| 90 | 6 cups | 7 cups | 8 cups |
| 100 | 6 1/2 cups | 7 1/2 cups | 8 1/2 cups |

## Recipe 5: Cod & Carrot Feast

**Ingredients (for 1 cup):**

- 1 oz cod (30g)
- 2 tbsp quinoa, cooked (20g)
- 1/2 cup kale, chopped (60g)
- 1/2 cup carrots, chopped (60g)
- 1/3 cup apples, chopped (40g)
- 1/2 tsp olive oil (2.5g)
- 1 cup water

**Preparation Time:**

- **Prep Time**: 10 minutes
- **Cook Time**: 4 hours
- **Total Time**: 4 hours 10 minutes
- **Difficulty Level**: Easy

## Instructions:

1. **Prepare the Ingredients**:
    - Cook the quinoa according to package instructions.
    - Chop the kale, carrots, and apples.
    - Cut the cod into small pieces.
2. **Combine in the Slow Cooker**:
    - Place the cod, quinoa, kale, carrots, and apples in the slow cooker.
    - Add olive oil and water.
3. **Cook**:
    - Set the slow cooker to low and cook for 4 hours or until the vegetables are tender and the cod is fully cooked.
4. **Cool and Serve**:
    - Allow the mixture to cool to a safe temperature before serving.
    - Portion according to your dog's size and daily caloric needs.

## Nutritional Information (per serving):

| Nutrient | Quantity (per cup) | Daily Value (%) |
|---|---|---|
| Calories | 160 kcal | - |
| Protein | 0.53 oz (6.5 g) | 20% |
| Fat | 0.01 oz (3.0 g) | 15% |
| Carbohydrates | 0.88 oz (21.3 g) | 53% |
| Fiber | 0.02 oz (2.5 g) | 2.5% |

**Suggested Portions (Daily):**

| Dog Size (lbs) | Low Activity | Moderate Activity | High Activity |
| --- | --- | --- | --- |
| 5 | 1 cup | 1 1/4 cups | 1 1/2 cups |
| 10 | 1 1/2 cups | 2 cups | 2 1/2 cups |
| 20 | 2 1/2 cups | 3 cups | 3 1/2 cups |
| 30 | 3 cups | 4 cups | 4 1/2 cups |
| 40 | 3 1/2 cups | 4 1/2 cups | 5 cups |
| 50 | 4 cups | 5 cups | 6 cups |
| 60 | 4 1/2 cups | 5 1/2 cups | 6 1/2 cups |
| 70 | 5 cups | 6 cups | 7 cups |
| 80 | 5 1/2 cups | 6 1/2 cups | 7 1/2 cups |
| 90 | 6 cups | 7 cups | 8 cups |
| 100 | 6 1/2 cups | 7 1/2 cups | 8 1/2 cups |

# Tuna Recipes

### Recipe 1: Tuna & Veggie Feast

**Ingredients (for 1 cup):**

- 0.88 oz tuna (25g)
- 2 tbsp brown rice, cooked (25g)
- 1 cup broccoli, chopped (80g)
- 1/2 cup carrots, chopped (70g)
- 1/3 cup apples, chopped (30g)
- 1 tsp olive oil (5g)
- 1 cup water

### Preparation Time:

- **Prep Time**: 10 minutes
- **Cook Time**: 4 hours
- **Total Time**: 4 hours 10 minutes
- **Difficulty Level**: Easy

### Instructions:

1. **Prepare the Ingredients**:
    - Cook the brown rice according to package instructions.
    - Chop the broccoli, carrots, and apples.
    - Cut the tuna into small pieces.
2. **Combine in the Slow Cooker**:
    - Place the tuna, brown rice, broccoli, carrots, and apples in the slow cooker.
    - Add olive oil and water.
3. **Cook**:
    - Set the slow cooker to low and cook for 4 hours or until the vegetables are tender and the tuna is fully cooked.
4. **Cool and Serve**:
    - Allow the mixture to cool to a safe temperature before serving.
    - Portion according to your dog's size and daily caloric needs.

### Nutritional Information (per serving):

| Nutrient | Quantity (per cup) | Daily Value (%) |
|---|---|---|
| Calories | 179 kcal | - |
| Protein | 0.39 oz (11.2 g) | 27.8% |
| Fat | 0.01 oz (2.6 g) | 14.3% |
| Carbohydrates | 0.89 oz (25.7 g) | 57.9% |
| Fiber | 0.02 oz (2.0 g) | 2.0% |

## Suggested Portions (Daily):

| Dog Size (lbs) | Low Activity | Moderate Activity | High Activity |
|---|---|---|---|
| 5 | 1 cup | 1 1/4 cups | 1 1/2 cups |
| 10 | 1 1/2 cups | 2 cups | 2 1/2 cups |
| 20 | 2 1/2 cups | 3 cups | 3 1/2 cups |
| 30 | 3 cups | 4 cups | 4 1/2 cups |
| 40 | 3 1/2 cups | 4 1/2 cups | 5 cups |
| 50 | 4 cups | 5 cups | 6 cups |
| 60 | 4 1/2 cups | 5 1/2 cups | 6 1/2 cups |
| 70 | 5 cups | 6 cups | 7 cups |
| 80 | 5 1/2 cups | 6 1/2 cups | 7 1/2 cups |
| 90 | 6 cups | 7 cups | 8 cups |
| 100 | 6 1/2 cups | 7 1/2 cups | 8 1/2 cups |

## Recipe 2: Tuna & Green Bean Delight

**Ingredients (for 1 cup):**

- 0.77 oz tuna (22g)
- 2 tbsp brown rice, cooked (25g)
- 1 cup green beans, chopped (60g)
- 1/2 cup sweet potatoes, chopped (45g)
- 1/3 cup peas (20g)
- 1/2 tsp olive oil (3g)
- 1 cup water

### Preparation Time:

- **Prep Time**: 10 minutes
- **Cook Time**: 4 hours
- **Total Time**: 4 hours 10 minutes
- **Difficulty Level**: Easy

### Instructions:

1. **Prepare the Ingredients**:
   - Cook the brown rice according to package instructions.
   - Chop the green beans and sweet potatoes.
   - Measure out the peas.
   - Cut the tuna into small pieces.
2. **Combine in the Slow Cooker**:
   - Place the tuna, brown rice, green beans, sweet potatoes, and peas in the slow cooker.
   - Add olive oil and water.
3. **Cook**:
   - Set the slow cooker to low and cook for 4 hours or until the vegetables are tender and the tuna is fully cooked.

4. **Cool and Serve**:
    - Allow the mixture to cool to a safe temperature before serving.
    - Portion according to your dog's size and daily caloric needs.

## Nutritional Information (per serving):

| Nutrient | Quantity (per cup) | Daily Value (%) |
|---|---|---|
| Calories | 160 kcal | - |
| Protein | 0.27 oz (7.8 g) | 28.0% |
| Fat | 0.01 oz (1.5 g) | 9.3% |
| Carbohydrates | 0.88 oz (24.9 g) | 62.7% |
| Fiber | 0.02 oz (2.3 g) | 2.3% |

## Suggested Portions (Daily):

| Dog Size (lbs) | Low Activity | Moderate Activity | High Activity |
|---|---|---|---|
| 5 | 1 cup | 1 1/4 cups | 1 1/2 cups |
| 10 | 1 1/2 cups | 2 cups | 2 1/2 cups |
| 20 | 2 1/2 cups | 3 cups | 3 1/2 cups |
| 30 | 3 cups | 4 cups | 4 1/2 cups |
| 40 | 3 1/2 cups | 4 1/2 cups | 5 cups |
| 50 | 4 cups | 5 cups | 6 cups |
| 60 | 4 1/2 cups | 5 1/2 cups | 6 1/2 cups |
| 70 | 5 cups | 6 cups | 7 cups |
| 80 | 5 1/2 cups | 6 1/2 cups | 7 1/2 cups |
| 90 | 6 cups | 7 cups | 8 cups |
| 100 | 6 1/2 cups | 7 1/2 cups | 8 1/2 cups |

## Recipe 3: Tuna & Spinach Delight

**Ingredients (for 1 cup):**

- 0.77 oz tuna (22g)
- 2 tbsp brown rice, cooked (20g)
- 1/2 cup carrots, chopped (60g)
- 1/2 cup spinach, chopped (50g)
- 1/4 cup apples, chopped (25g)
- 1/2 tsp olive oil (2g)
- 1 cup water

**Preparation Time:**

- **Prep Time**: 10 minutes
- **Cook Time**: 4 hours
- **Total Time**: 4 hours 10 minutes
- **Difficulty Level**: Easy

**Instructions:**

1. **Prepare the Ingredients:**
   - Cook the brown rice according to package instructions.
   - Chop the carrots, spinach, and apples.
   - Cut the tuna into small pieces.
2. **Combine in the Slow Cooker:**
   - Place the tuna, brown rice, carrots, spinach, and apples in the slow cooker.
   - Add olive oil and water.
3. **Cook:**
   - Set the slow cooker to low and cook for 4 hours or until the vegetables are tender and the tuna is fully cooked.
4. **Cool and Serve:**
   - Allow the mixture to cool to a safe temperature before serving.
   - Portion according to your dog's size and daily caloric needs.

### Nutritional Information (per serving):

| Nutrient | Quantity (per cup) | Daily Value (%) |
|---|---|---|
| Calories | 159.8 kcal | - |
| Protein | 0.35 oz (9.9 g) | 27.6% |
| Fat | 0.01 oz (1.8 g) | 10.1% |
| Carbohydrates | 0.87 oz (24.5 g) | 57.4% |
| Fiber | 0.02 oz (2.1 g) | 2.1% |

### Suggested Portions (Daily):

| Dog Size (lbs) | Low Activity | Moderate Activity | High Activity |
|---|---|---|---|
| 5 | 1 cup | 1 1/4 cups | 1 1/2 cups |
| 10 | 1 1/2 cups | 2 cups | 2 1/2 cups |
| 20 | 2 1/2 cups | 3 cups | 3 1/2 cups |
| 30 | 3 cups | 4 cups | 4 1/2 cups |
| 40 | 3 1/2 cups | 4 1/2 cups | 5 cups |
| 50 | 4 cups | 5 cups | 6 cups |
| 60 | 4 1/2 cups | 5 1/2 cups | 6 1/2 cups |
| 70 | 5 cups | 6 cups | 7 cups |
| 80 | 5 1/2 cups | 6 1/2 cups | 7 1/2 cups |
| 90 | 6 cups | 7 cups | 8 cups |
| 100 | 6 1/2 cups | 7 1/2 cups | 8 1/2 cups |

### Recipe 4: Tuna & Broccoli Delight

**Ingredients (for 1 cup):**

- 1 oz tuna (28g)
- 2 tbsp brown rice, cooked (25g)
- 1/2 cup broccoli, chopped (60g)
- 1/3 cup pumpkin, cooked and mashed (50g)

- 1/4 cup blueberries, chopped (30g)
- 1 tsp olive oil (4g)
- 1 cup water

**Preparation Time:**

- **Prep Time**: 10 minutes
- **Cook Time**: 4 hours
- **Total Time**: 4 hours 10 minutes
- **Difficulty Level**: Easy

**Instructions:**

1. **Prepare the Ingredients**:
    - Cook the brown rice according to package instructions.
    - Chop the broccoli and blueberries.
    - Cook and mash the pumpkin.
    - Cut the tuna into small pieces.
2. **Combine in the Slow Cooker**:
    - Place the tuna, brown rice, broccoli, pumpkin, and blueberries in the slow cooker.
    - Add olive oil and water.
3. **Cook**:
    - Set the slow cooker to low and cook for 4 hours or until the vegetables are tender and the tuna is fully cooked.
4. **Cool and Serve**:
    - Allow the mixture to cool to a safe temperature before serving.
    - Portion according to your dog's size and daily caloric needs.

## Nutritional Information (per serving):

| Nutrient | Quantity (per cup) | Daily Value (%) |
|---|---|---|
| Calories | 160 kcal | - |
| Protein | 0.28 oz (7.9 g) | 27.5% |
| Fat | 0.02 oz (1.8 g) | 10.1% |
| Carbohydrates | 0.81 oz (22.9 g) | 57.1% |
| Fiber | 0.03 oz (2.1 g) | 2.6% |

## Suggested Portions (Daily):

| Dog Size (lbs) | Low Activity | Moderate Activity | High Activity |
|---|---|---|---|
| 5 | 1 cup | 1 1/4 cups | 1 1/2 cups |
| 10 | 1 1/2 cups | 2 cups | 2 1/2 cups |
| 20 | 2 1/2 cups | 3 cups | 3 1/2 cups |
| 30 | 3 cups | 4 cups | 4 1/2 cups |
| 40 | 3 1/2 cups | 4 1/2 cups | 5 cups |
| 50 | 4 cups | 5 cups | 6 cups |
| 60 | 4 1/2 cups | 5 1/2 cups | 6 1/2 cups |
| 70 | 5 cups | 6 cups | 7 cups |
| 80 | 5 1/2 cups | 6 1/2 cups | 7 1/2 cups |
| 90 | 6 cups | 7 cups | 8 cups |
| 100 | 6 1/2 cups | 7 1/2 cups | 8 1/2 cups |

## Recipe 5: Tuna & Sweet Potato Feast

**Ingredients (for 1 cup):**

- 1 oz tuna (28g)
- 2 tbsp quinoa, cooked (20g)
- 1/2 cup sweet potatoes, diced (50g)
- 1/3 cup green beans, chopped (50g)
- 1/4 cup apples, chopped (30g)
- 1 tsp coconut oil (4g)
- 1 cup water

**Preparation Time:**

- **Prep Time**: 10 minutes
- **Cook Time**: 4 hours
- **Total Time**: 4 hours 10 minutes
- **Difficulty Level**: Easy

**Instructions:**

1. **Prepare the Ingredients**:
    - Cook the quinoa according to package instructions.
    - Dice the sweet potatoes and apples.
    - Chop the green beans.
    - Cut the tuna into small pieces.
2. **Combine in the Slow Cooker**:
    - Place the tuna, quinoa, sweet potatoes, green beans, and apples in the slow cooker.
    - Add coconut oil and water.
3. **Cook**:
    - Set the slow cooker to low and cook for 4 hours or until the vegetables are tender and the tuna is fully cooked.

4. **Cool and Serve**:
    - Allow the mixture to cool to a safe temperature before serving.
    - Portion according to your dog's size and daily caloric needs.

**Nutritional Information (per serving):**

| Nutrient | Quantity (per cup) | Daily Value (%) |
|---|---|---|
| Calories | 160 kcal | - |
| Protein | 0.28 oz (7.9 g) | 27.5% |
| Fat | 0.02 oz (1.8 g) | 10.1% |
| Carbohydrates | 0.81 oz (22.9 g) | 57.1% |
| Fiber | 0.03 oz (2.1 g) | 2.6% |

**Suggested Portions (Daily):**

| Dog Size (lbs) | Low Activity | Moderate Activity | High Activity |
|---|---|---|---|
| 5 | 1 cup | 1 1/4 cups | 1 1/2 cups |
| 10 | 1 1/2 cups | 2 cups | 2 1/2 cups |
| 20 | 2 1/2 cups | 3 cups | 3 1/2 cups |
| 30 | 3 cups | 4 cups | 4 1/2 cups |
| 40 | 3 1/2 cups | 4 1/2 cups | 5 cups |
| 50 | 4 cups | 5 cups | 6 cups |
| 60 | 4 1/2 cups | 5 1/2 cups | 6 1/2 cups |
| 70 | 5 cups | 6 cups | 7 cups |
| 80 | 5 1/2 cups | 6 1/2 cups | 7 1/2 cups |
| 90 | 6 cups | 7 cups | 8 cups |
| 100 | 6 1/2 cups | 7 1/2 cups | 8 1/2 cups |

# Sardine Recipes

### Recipe 1: Sardine & Veggie Medley

**Ingredients (for 1 cup):**

- 1.06 oz sardines (30g)
- 2 tbsp brown rice, cooked (25g)
- 1/2 cup carrots, chopped (50g)
- 1/2 cup zucchini, chopped (50g)
- 1/4 cup peas (30g)
- 1/2 tsp olive oil (2g)
- 1 cup water

**Preparation Time:**

- **Prep Time**: 10 minutes
- **Cook Time**: 4 hours
- **Total Time**: 4 hours 10 minutes
- **Difficulty Level**: Easy

**Instructions:**

1. **Prepare the Ingredients**:
    - Cook the brown rice according to package instructions.
    - Chop the carrots and zucchini.
    - Measure out the peas.
    - Cut the sardines into small pieces.
2. **Combine in the Slow Cooker**:
    - Place the sardines, brown rice, carrots, zucchini, and peas in the slow cooker.
    - Add olive oil and water.
3. **Cook**:
    - Set the slow cooker to low and cook for 4 hours or until the vegetables are tender and the sardines are fully cooked.
4. **Cool and Serve**:
    - Allow the mixture to cool to a safe temperature before serving.
    - Portion according to your dog's size and daily caloric needs.

### Nutritional Information (per serving):

| Nutrient | Quantity (per cup) | Daily Value (%) |
|---|---|---|
| Calories | 164.13 kcal | - |
| Protein | 0.37 oz (10.4 g) | 31.8% |
| Fat | 0.02 oz (1.9 g) | 17.4% |
| Carbohydrates | 0.82 oz (23.9 g) | 50.8% |
| Fiber | 0.02 oz (1.8 g) | 1.8% |

## Suggested Portions (Daily):

| Dog Size (lbs) | Low Activity | Moderate Activity | High Activity |
|---|---|---|---|
| 5 | 1 cup | 1 1/4 cups | 1 1/2 cups |
| 10 | 1 1/2 cups | 2 cups | 2 1/2 cups |
| 20 | 2 1/2 cups | 3 cups | 3 1/2 cups |
| 30 | 3 cups | 4 cups | 4 1/2 cups |
| 40 | 3 1/2 cups | 4 1/2 cups | 5 cups |
| 50 | 4 cups | 5 cups | 6 cups |
| 60 | 4 1/2 cups | 5 1/2 cups | 6 1/2 cups |
| 70 | 5 cups | 6 cups | 7 cups |
| 80 | 5 1/2 cups | 6 1/2 cups | 7 1/2 cups |
| 90 | 6 cups | 7 cups | 8 cups |
| 100 | 6 1/2 cups | 7 1/2 cups | 8 1/2 cups |

## Recipe 2: Sardine & Sweet Potato Feast

**Ingredients (for 1 cup):**

- 0.88 oz sardines (25g)
- 2 tbsp quinoa, cooked (20g)
- 1/2 cup sweet potatoes, diced (50g)
- 1/2 cup green beans, chopped (50g)
- 1/4 cup apples, chopped (30g)
- 1/2 tsp olive oil (2g)
- 1 cup water

**Preparation Time:**

- **Prep Time**: 10 minutes
- **Cook Time**: 4 hours
- **Total Time**: 4 hours 10 minutes
- **Difficulty Level**: Easy

**Instructions:**

1. **Prepare the Ingredients**:
    - Cook the quinoa according to package instructions.
    - Dice the sweet potatoes and apples.
    - Chop the green beans.
    - Cut the sardines into small pieces.
2. **Combine in the Slow Cooker**:
    - Place the sardines, quinoa, sweet potatoes, green beans, and apples in the slow cooker.
    - Add olive oil and water.
3. **Cook**:
    - Set the slow cooker to low and cook for 4 hours or until the vegetables are tender and the sardines are fully cooked.

4. **Cool and Serve**:
    o Allow the mixture to cool to a safe temperature before serving.
    o Portion according to your dog's size and daily caloric needs.

## Nutritional Information (per serving):

| Nutrient | Quantity (per cup) | Daily Value (%) |
|---|---|---|
| Calories | 167.78 kcal | - |
| Protein | 0.35 oz (9.8 g) | 24.9% |
| Fat | 0.02 oz (2.5 g) | 14.9% |
| Carbohydrates | 0.92 oz (25.5 g) | 60.1% |
| Fiber | 0.02 oz (2.0 g) | 2.0% |

## Suggested Portions (Daily):

| Dog Size (lbs) | Low Activity | Moderate Activity | High Activity |
|---|---|---|---|
| 5 | 1 cup | 1 1/4 cups | 1 1/2 cups |
| 10 | 1 1/2 cups | 2 cups | 2 1/2 cups |
| 20 | 2 1/2 cups | 3 cups | 3 1/2 cups |
| 30 | 3 cups | 4 cups | 4 1/2 cups |
| 40 | 3 1/2 cups | 4 1/2 cups | 5 cups |
| 50 | 4 cups | 5 cups | 6 cups |
| 60 | 4 1/2 cups | 5 1/2 cups | 6 1/2 cups |
| 70 | 5 cups | 6 cups | 7 cups |
| 80 | 5 1/2 cups | 6 1/2 cups | 7 1/2 cups |
| 90 | 6 cups | 7 cups | 8 cups |
| 100 | 6 1/2 cups | 7 1/2 cups | 8 1/2 cups |

## Recipe 3: Sardine & Pumpkin Delight

**Ingredients (for 1 cup):**

- 0.70 oz sardines (20g)
- 1.5 tbsp oats, cooked (15g)
- 1/2 cup spinach, chopped (60g)
- 1/2 cup pumpkin, cooked and mashed (50g)
- 1/4 cup blueberries, chopped (30g)
- 1/2 tsp olive oil (2g)
- 1 cup water

**Preparation Time:**

- **Prep Time**: 10 minutes
- **Cook Time**: 4 hours
- **Total Time**: 4 hours 10 minutes
- **Difficulty Level**: Easy

**Instructions:**

1. **Prepare the Ingredients:**
   - Cook the oats according to package instructions.
   - Chop the spinach and blueberries.
   - Cook and mash the pumpkin.
   - Cut the sardines into small pieces.
2. **Combine in the Slow Cooker:**
   - Place the sardines, oats, spinach, pumpkin, and blueberries in the slow cooker.
   - Add olive oil and water.
3. **Cook:**
   - Set the slow cooker to low and cook for 4 hours or until the vegetables are tender and the sardines are fully cooked.
4. **Cool and Serve:**
   - Allow the mixture to cool to a safe temperature before serving.
   - Portion according to your dog's size and daily caloric needs.

## Nutritional Information (per serving):

| Nutrient | Quantity (per cup) | Daily Value (%) |
|---|---|---|
| Calories | 161.53 kcal | - |
| Protein | 0.28 oz (8.1 g) | 28.0% |
| Fat | 0.02 oz (2.6 g) | 16.2% |
| Carbohydrates | 0.88 oz (22.5 g) | 55.8% |
| Fiber | 0.02 oz (2.0 g) | 2.0% |

## Suggested Portions (Daily):

| Dog Size (lbs) | Low Activity | Moderate Activity | High Activity |
|---|---|---|---|
| 5 | 1 cup | 1 1/4 cups | 1 1/2 cups |
| 10 | 1 1/2 cups | 2 cups | 2 1/2 cups |
| 20 | 2 1/2 cups | 3 cups | 3 1/2 cups |
| 30 | 3 cups | 4 cups | 4 1/2 cups |
| 40 | 3 1/2 cups | 4 1/2 cups | 5 cups |
| 50 | 4 cups | 5 cups | 6 cups |
| 60 | 4 1/2 cups | 5 1/2 cups | 6 1/2 cups |
| 70 | 5 cups | 6 cups | 7 cups |
| 80 | 5 1/2 cups | 6 1/2 cups | 7 1/2 cups |
| 90 | 6 cups | 7 cups | 8 cups |
| 100 | 6 1/2 cups | 7 1/2 cups | 8 1/2 cups |

## Recipe 4: Sardine & Kale Delight

**Ingredients (for 1 cup):**

- 0.88 oz sardines (25g)
- 2 tbsp brown rice, cooked (20g)
- 1/2 cup kale, chopped (50g)

- 1/2 cup carrots, chopped (50g)
- 1/4 cup strawberries, chopped (30g)
- 1/2 tsp olive oil (2g)
- 1 cup water

**Preparation Time:**

- **Prep Time**: 10 minutes
- **Cook Time**: 4 hours
- **Total Time**: 4 hours 10 minutes
- **Difficulty Level**: Easy

**Instructions:**

1. **Prepare the Ingredients**:
    - Cook the brown rice according to package instructions.
    - Chop the kale, carrots, and strawberries.
    - Cut the sardines into small pieces.
2. **Combine in the Slow Cooker**:
    - Place the sardines, brown rice, kale, carrots, and strawberries in the slow cooker.
    - Add olive oil and water.
3. **Cook**:
    - Set the slow cooker to low and cook for 4 hours or until the vegetables are tender and the sardines are fully cooked.
4. **Cool and Serve**:
    - Allow the mixture to cool to a safe temperature before serving.
    - Portion according to your dog's size and daily caloric needs.

## Nutritional Information (per serving):

| Nutrient | Quantity (per cup) | Daily Value (%) |
|---|---|---|
| Calories | 160 kcal | - |
| Protein | 0.34 oz (9.5 g) | 27.6% |
| Fat | 0.02 oz (2.6 g) | 14.6% |
| Carbohydrates | 0.83 oz (23.2 g) | 55.7% |
| Fiber | 0.02 oz (2.2 g) | 2.2% |

## Suggested Portions (Daily):

| Dog Size (lbs) | Low Activity | Moderate Activity | High Activity |
|---|---|---|---|
| 5 | 1 cup | 1 1/4 cups | 1 1/2 cups |
| 10 | 1 1/2 cups | 2 cups | 2 1/2 cups |
| 20 | 2 1/2 cups | 3 cups | 3 1/2 cups |
| 30 | 3 cups | 4 cups | 4 1/2 cups |
| 40 | 3 1/2 cups | 4 1/2 cups | 5 cups |
| 50 | 4 cups | 5 cups | 6 cups |
| 60 | 4 1/2 cups | 5 1/2 cups | 6 1/2 cups |
| 70 | 5 cups | 6 cups | 7 cups |
| 80 | 5 1/2 cups | 6 1/2 cups | 7 1/2 cups |
| 90 | 6 cups | 7 cups | 8 cups |
| 100 | 6 1/2 cups | 7 1/2 cups | 8 1/2 cups |

## Recipe 5: Sardine & Spinach Delight

**Ingredients (for 1 cup):**

- 1 oz sardine (30g)
- 2 tbsp brown rice, cooked (20g)
- 3/4 cup spinach, chopped (75g)
- 1/2 cup carrots, chopped (50g)
- 1/3 cup blueberries, chopped (40g)
- 1/2 tsp olive oil (2g)
- 1 cup water

**Preparation Time:**

- **Prep Time**: 10 minutes
- **Cook Time**: 4 hours
- **Total Time**: 4 hours 10 minutes
- **Difficulty Level**: Easy

**Instructions:**

1. **Prepare the Ingredients**:
   - Cook the brown rice according to package instructions.
   - Chop the spinach, carrots, and blueberries.
   - Cut the sardine into small pieces.
2. **Combine in the Slow Cooker**:
   - Place the sardine, brown rice, spinach, carrots, and blueberries in the slow cooker.
   - Add olive oil and water.
3. **Cook**:
   - Set the slow cooker to low and cook for 4 hours or until the vegetables are tender and the sardine is fully cooked.
4. **Cool and Serve**:
   - Allow the mixture to cool to a safe temperature before serving.

- Portion according to your dog's size and daily caloric needs.

## Nutritional Information (per serving):

| Nutrient | Quantity (per cup) | Daily Value (%) |
|---|---|---|
| Calories | 160 kcal | - |
| Protein | 0.38 oz (10.8 g) | 27% |
| Fat | 0.02 oz (2.3 g) | 13% |
| Carbohydrates | 0.98 oz (27.8 g) | 57% |
| Fiber | 0.03 oz (2.4 g) | 2.4% |

## Suggested Portions (Daily):

| Dog Size (lbs) | Low Activity | Moderate Activity | High Activity |
|---|---|---|---|
| 5 | 1 cup | 1 1/4 cups | 1 1/2 cups |
| 10 | 1 1/2 cups | 2 cups | 2 1/2 cups |
| 20 | 2 1/2 cups | 3 cups | 3 1/2 cups |
| 30 | 3 cups | 4 cups | 4 1/2 cups |
| 40 | 3 1/2 cups | 4 1/2 cups | 5 cups |
| 50 | 4 cups | 5 cups | 6 cups |
| 60 | 4 1/2 cups | 5 1/2 cups | 6 1/2 cups |
| 70 | 5 cups | 6 cups | 7 cups |
| 80 | 5 1/2 cups | 6 1/2 cups | 7 1/2 cups |
| 90 | 6 cups | 7 cups | 8 cups |
| 100 | 6 1/2 cups | 7 1/2 cups | 8 1/2 cups |

# Trout Recipes

### Recipe 1: Trout & Veggie Mix

**Ingredients (for 1 cup):**

- 1 oz trout (30g)
- 2 tbsp quinoa, cooked (30g)
- 1/2 cup spinach, chopped (50g)
- 1/2 cup carrots, chopped (50g)
- 1/4 cup apples, chopped (30g)
- 1/2 tsp olive oil (2g)
- 1 cup water

**Preparation Time:**

- **Prep Time**: 10 minutes
- **Cook Time**: 4 hours
- **Total Time**: 4 hours 10 minutes
- **Difficulty Level**: Easy

**Instructions:**

1. **Prepare the Ingredients**:
    - Cook the quinoa according to package instructions.
    - Chop the spinach, carrots, and apples.
    - Cut the trout into small pieces.
2. **Combine in the Slow Cooker**:
    - Place the trout, quinoa, spinach, carrots, and apples in the slow cooker.
    - Add olive oil and water.
3. **Cook**:
    - Set the slow cooker to low and cook for 4 hours or until the vegetables are tender and the trout is fully cooked.
4. **Cool and Serve**:
    - Allow the mixture to cool to a safe temperature before serving.
    - Portion according to your dog's size and daily caloric needs.

### Nutritional Information (per serving):

| Nutrient | Quantity (per cup) | Daily Value (%) |
|---|---|---|
| Calories | 160 kcal | - |
| Protein | 0.37 oz (10.4 g) | 26% |
| Fat | 0.02 oz (2.6 g) | 14.6% |
| Carbohydrates | 0.87 oz (24.6 g) | 57.4% |
| Fiber | 0.02 oz (2.2 g) | 2.2% |

## Suggested Portions (Daily):

| Dog Size (lbs) | Low Activity | Moderate Activity | High Activity |
|---|---|---|---|
| 5 | 1 cup | 1 1/4 cups | 1 1/2 cups |
| 10 | 1 1/2 cups | 2 cups | 2 1/2 cups |
| 20 | 2 1/2 cups | 3 cups | 3 1/2 cups |
| 30 | 3 cups | 4 cups | 4 1/2 cups |
| 40 | 3 1/2 cups | 4 1/2 cups | 5 cups |
| 50 | 4 cups | 5 cups | 6 cups |
| 60 | 4 1/2 cups | 5 1/2 cups | 6 1/2 cups |
| 70 | 5 cups | 6 cups | 7 cups |
| 80 | 5 1/2 cups | 6 1/2 cups | 7 1/2 cups |
| 90 | 6 cups | 7 cups | 8 cups |
| 100 | 6 1/2 cups | 7 1/2 cups | 8 1/2 cups |

## Recipe 2: Trout & Sweet Potato Medley

**Ingredients (for 1 cup):**

- 0.88 oz trout (25g)
- 1 tbsp brown rice, cooked (15g)
- 1/2 cup broccoli, chopped (50g)
- 1/2 cup sweet potatoes, diced (50g)
- 1/4 cup blueberries, chopped (30g)
- 1/2 tsp olive oil (2g)
- 1 cup water

**Preparation Time:**

- **Prep Time**: 10 minutes
- **Cook Time**: 4 hours
- **Total Time**: 4 hours 10 minutes
- **Difficulty Level**: Easy

**Instructions:**

1. **Prepare the Ingredients**:
    - Cook the brown rice according to package instructions.
    - Chop the broccoli and blueberries.
    - Dice the sweet potatoes.
    - Cut the trout into small pieces.
2. **Combine in the Slow Cooker**:
    - Place the trout, brown rice, broccoli, sweet potatoes, and blueberries in the slow cooker.
    - Add olive oil and water.
3. **Cook**:
    - Set the slow cooker to low and cook for 4 hours or until the vegetables are tender and the trout is fully cooked.

4. **Cool and Serve**:
    - Allow the mixture to cool to a safe temperature before serving.
    - Portion according to your dog's size and daily caloric needs.

## Nutritional Information (per serving):

| Nutrient | Quantity (per cup) | Daily Value (%) |
|---|---|---|
| Calories | 160 kcal | - |
| Protein | 0.32 oz (9.1 g) | 22.8% |
| Fat | 0.02 oz (2.1 g) | 11.7% |
| Carbohydrates | 0.93 oz (26.2 g) | 65.5% |
| Fiber | 0.02 oz (2.2 g) | 2.2% |

## Suggested Portions (Daily):

| Dog Size (lbs) | Low Activity | Moderate Activity | High Activity |
|---|---|---|---|
| 5 | 1 cup | 1 1/4 cups | 1 1/2 cups |
| 10 | 1 1/2 cups | 2 cups | 2 1/2 cups |
| 20 | 2 1/2 cups | 3 cups | 3 1/2 cups |
| 30 | 3 cups | 4 cups | 4 1/2 cups |
| 40 | 3 1/2 cups | 4 1/2 cups | 5 cups |
| 50 | 4 cups | 5 cups | 6 cups |
| 60 | 4 1/2 cups | 5 1/2 cups | 6 1/2 cups |
| 70 | 5 cups | 6 cups | 7 cups |
| 80 | 5 1/2 cups | 6 1/2 cups | 7 1/2 cups |
| 90 | 6 cups | 7 cups | 8 cups |
| 100 | 6 1/2 cups | 7 1/2 cups | 8 1/2 cups |

## Recipe 3: Trout & Veggie Delight

**Ingredients (for 1 cup):**

- 0.88 oz trout (25g)
- 1 tbsp oats, cooked (15g)
- 1/2 cup green beans, chopped (50g)
- 1/2 cup sweet potatoes, diced (50g)
- 1/4 cup apples, chopped (30g)
- 1/2 tsp olive oil (2g)
- 1 cup water

**Preparation Time:**

- **Prep Time**: 10 minutes
- **Cook Time**: 4 hours
- **Total Time**: 4 hours 10 minutes
- **Difficulty Level**: Easy

**Instructions:**

1. **Prepare the Ingredients**:
   - Cook the oats according to package instructions.
   - Chop the green beans and apples.
   - Dice the sweet potatoes.
   - Cut the trout into small pieces.
2. **Combine in the Slow Cooker**:
   - Place the trout, oats, green beans, sweet potatoes, and apples in the slow cooker.
   - Add olive oil and water.
3. **Cook**:
   - Set the slow cooker to low and cook for 4 hours or until the vegetables are tender and the trout is fully cooked.
4. **Cool and Serve**:
   - Allow the mixture to cool to a safe temperature before serving.
   - Portion according to your dog's size and daily caloric needs.

## Nutritional Information (per serving):

| Nutrient | Quantity (per cup) | Daily Value (%) |
|---|---|---|
| Calories | 160 kcal | - |
| Protein | 0.32 oz (9.1 g) | 23% |
| Fat | 0.02 oz (2.1 g) | 12% |
| Carbohydrates | 0.93 oz (26.2 g) | 65% |
| Fiber | 0.02 oz (2.2 g) | 2.2% |

## Suggested Portions (Daily):

| Dog Size (lbs) | Low Activity | Moderate Activity | High Activity |
|---|---|---|---|
| 5 | 1 cup | 1 1/4 cups | 1 1/2 cups |
| 10 | 1 1/2 cups | 2 cups | 2 1/2 cups |
| 20 | 2 1/2 cups | 3 cups | 3 1/2 cups |
| 30 | 3 cups | 4 cups | 4 1/2 cups |
| 40 | 3 1/2 cups | 4 1/2 cups | 5 cups |
| 50 | 4 cups | 5 cups | 6 cups |
| 60 | 4 1/2 cups | 5 1/2 cups | 6 1/2 cups |
| 70 | 5 cups | 6 cups | 7 cups |
| 80 | 5 1/2 cups | 6 1/2 cups | 7 1/2 cups |
| 90 | 6 cups | 7 cups | 8 cups |
| 100 | 6 1/2 cups | 7 1/2 cups | 8 1/2 cups |

# Recipe 4: Trout & Carrot Fiesta

**Ingredients (for 1 cup):**

- 0.88 oz trout (25g)
- 1 tbsp quinoa, cooked (15g)
- 1/2 cup carrots, chopped (50g)
- 1/2 cup peas (50g)
- 1/4 cup strawberries, chopped (30g)
- 1/2 tsp olive oil (2g)
- 1 cup water

**Preparation Time:**

- **Prep Time**: 10 minutes
- **Cook Time**: 4 hours
- **Total Time**: 4 hours 10 minutes
- **Difficulty Level**: Easy

**Instructions:**

1. **Prepare the Ingredients**:
    - Cook the quinoa according to package instructions.
    - Chop the carrots and strawberries.
    - Measure out the peas.
    - Cut the trout into small pieces.
2. **Combine in the Slow Cooker**:
    - Place the trout, quinoa, carrots, peas, and strawberries in the slow cooker.
    - Add olive oil and water.
3. **Cook**:
    - Set the slow cooker to low and cook for 4 hours or until the vegetables are tender and the trout is fully cooked.
4. **Cool and Serve**:
    - Allow the mixture to cool to a safe temperature before serving.
    - Portion according to your dog's size and daily caloric needs.

## Nutritional Information (per serving):

| Nutrient | Quantity (per cup) | Daily Value (%) |
|---|---|---|
| Calories | 160 kcal | - |
| Protein | 0.32 oz (9.1 g) | 23% |
| Fat | 0.02 oz (2.1 g) | 12% |
| Carbohydrates | 0.93 oz (26.2 g) | 65% |
| Fiber | 0.02 oz (2.2 g) | 2.2% |

## Suggested Portions (Daily):

| Dog Size (lbs) | Low Activity | Moderate Activity | High Activity |
|---|---|---|---|
| 5 | 1 cup | 1 1/4 cups | 1 1/2 cups |
| 10 | 1 1/2 cups | 2 cups | 2 1/2 cups |
| 20 | 2 1/2 cups | 3 cups | 3 1/2 cups |
| 30 | 3 cups | 4 cups | 4 1/2 cups |
| 40 | 3 1/2 cups | 4 1/2 cups | 5 cups |
| 50 | 4 cups | 5 cups | 6 cups |
| 60 | 4 1/2 cups | 5 1/2 cups | 6 1/2 cups |
| 70 | 5 cups | 6 cups | 7 cups |
| 80 | 5 1/2 cups | 6 1/2 cups | 7 1/2 cups |
| 90 | 6 cups | 7 cups | 8 cups |
| 100 | 6 1/2 cups | 7 1/2 cups | 8 1/2 cups |

## Recipe 5: Trout & Pumpkin Harvest

**Ingredients (for 1 cup):**

- 1.05 oz trout (30g)
- 2 tbsp brown rice, cooked (20g)
- 1/2 cup zucchini, chopped (50g)
- 1/2 cup pumpkin, cooked and diced (50g)
- 1/3 cup blueberries, chopped (40g)
- 1/2 tsp olive oil (2g)
- 1 cup water

**Preparation Time:**

- **Prep Time**: 10 minutes
- **Cook Time**: 4 hours
- **Total Time**: 4 hours 10 minutes
- **Difficulty Level**: Easy

**Instructions:**

1. **Prepare the Ingredients**:
    - Cook the brown rice according to package instructions.
    - Chop the zucchini, pumpkin, and blueberries.
    - Cut the trout into small pieces.
2. **Combine in the Slow Cooker**:
    - Place the trout, brown rice, zucchini, pumpkin, and blueberries in the slow cooker.
    - Add olive oil and water.
3. **Cook**:
    - Set the slow cooker to low and cook for 4 hours or until the vegetables are tender and the trout is fully cooked.
4. **Cool and Serve**:
    - Allow the mixture to cool to a safe temperature before serving.
    - Portion according to your dog's size and daily caloric needs.

## Nutritional Information (per serving):

| Nutrient | Quantity (per cup) | Daily Value (%) |
|---|---|---|
| Calories | 160 kcal | - |
| Protein | 0.38 oz (10.8 g) | 27% |
| Fat | 0.02 oz (2.2 g) | 12% |
| Carbohydrates | 0.98 oz (27.8 g) | 60% |
| Fiber | 0.02 oz (1.5 g) | 1.5% |

## Suggested Portions (Daily):

| Dog Size (lbs) | Low Activity | Moderate Activity | High Activity |
|---|---|---|---|
| 5 | 1 cup | 1 1/4 cups | 1 1/2 cups |
| 10 | 1 1/2 cups | 2 cups | 2 1/2 cups |
| 20 | 2 1/2 cups | 3 cups | 3 1/2 cups |
| 30 | 3 cups | 4 cups | 4 1/2 cups |
| 40 | 3 1/2 cups | 4 1/2 cups | 5 cups |
| 50 | 4 cups | 5 cups | 6 cups |
| 60 | 4 1/2 cups | 5 1/2 cups | 6 1/2 cups |
| 70 | 5 cups | 6 cups | 7 cups |
| 80 | 5 1/2 cups | 6 1/2 cups | 7 1/2 cups |
| 90 | 6 cups | 7 cups | 8 cups |
| 100 | 6 1/2 cups | 7 1/2 cups | 8 1/2 cups |

# Bonus

Thank you so much for choosing "The Slow Cooker Dog Food Cookbook"!

Your dedication to providing the best nutrition for your dog shows just how much love and care you have for your furry friend. I am truly honored that you have decided to embark on this journey with me.

As a token of my appreciation, I am excited to offer you 4 exclusive bonuses for free:
1. Identifying and Managing Food Sensitivities
2. Managing Obesity in Dogs
3. Nutritional Needs of Senior Dogs
4. "Pawsitively Delicious: 10 DIY Summer Snacks for Dogs"

To receive these bonuses, simply send an email to: **gisellerayne.contact@gmail.com** and you'll get the material delivered right to your inbox.

Your opinion means the world to me. I invite you to share an honest review on Amazon. Your feedback will help other dog lovers discover this book and enhance the lives of their furry companions.

Thank you again for allowing me to be a part of your dog's care and happiness. Together, we can make a difference.

With deep gratitude,

Gisèlle Rayne

# Cooking Measurement Table

| U.S. Unit | Metric Equivalent | Notes |
| --- | --- | --- |
| **Weight** | | |
| 1 pound (lb) | 0.45 kilograms (kg) | Used for measuring meat |
| 1 ounce (oz) | 28.35 grams (g) | Used for small quantities of solids |
| **Volume (Liquids and Dry Ingredients)** | | |
| 1 cup | 240 milliliters (ml) | Used for liquids and dry ingredients |
| 1/2 cup | 120 milliliters (ml) | |
| 1/3 cup | 80 milliliters (ml) | |
| 1/4 cup | 60 milliliters (ml) | |
| **Small Volume Measurements** | | |
| 1 tablespoon (tbsp) | 15 milliliters (ml) | Used for small amounts of liquids and dry ingredients |
| 1 teaspoon (tsp) | 5 milliliters (ml) | Used for small amounts of liquids and dry ingredients |

# Conclusions

The journey explored through this book has provided a detailed and in-depth look at the importance of canine nutrition, highlighting the benefits of preparing homemade meals using the slow cooking technique. The combination of high-quality proteins, fresh vegetables, nutritious grains, and functional ingredients has proven to be an effective solution for enhancing the overall health and well-being of our four-legged friends. The nutritional approach presented here not only ensures a balanced and complete diet but also allows for the customization of meals based on the specific needs of each dog. This level of personalization is crucial for managing particular conditions such as food allergies, digestive sensitivities, joint problems, and other common canine ailments. Adopting fresh and natural ingredients, combined with proper preservation techniques, ensures that each meal is rich in essential nutrients and free from harmful additives. The recipes provided not only offer variety and flavor but also optimal nutritional intake that supports long-term canine health. Emerging trends in canine nutrition, such as the use of functional foods, eco-sustainable ingredients, and the integration of health-monitoring technologies, offer new opportunities to further improve the well-being of our pets. These innovations represent the future of canine nutrition, promoting an increasingly conscious and scientific approach to caring for our dogs.

In conclusion, preparing homemade meals for dogs is not only an act of love but a commitment to their health and happiness. By implementing the practices and recipes shared in this book, we can ensure our dogs live longer, healthier, and more fulfilling lives, strengthening the special bond we share with them.

Made in the USA
Las Vegas, NV
15 June 2025